Martial Arts for Women

A Practical Guide

Martial Arts for Women

A Practical Guide

by

Jennifer Lawler

Turtle Press   **Hartford, CT**

Martial Arts for Women: A Practical Guide

To contact the author or order additional copies of this book:
Turtle Press
401 Silas Deane Hwy.
PO Box 290206
Wethersfield, CT 06129-0206
1-800-778-8785

ISBN   1-880336-16-2
First Edition
Library of Congress Number 97-27231

Cataloging in Publication data

Lawler, Jennifer, 1965-
      Martial arts for women : a practical guide for women / by Jennifer
  Lawler. -- 1st ed.
         p. cm.
      Includes index.
      ISBN 1-880336-16-2
      1. Self-defense for women. 2. Martial arts. I Title
  GV1111.5.L391998
  796.8'082--dc21   97-27231

NOTE TO READERS

Consult a physician before undertaking this or any other exercise regimen. Neither the author nor the publisher assumes any responsibility for the use or misuse of the information contained in this book.

Contents

Introduction

When I first began my martial arts training, I was twenty-seven years old, out of shape, overweight, and suffering daily from the nearly crippling effects of rheumatoid arthritis. Suffice it to say that I did not have a healthy relationship with my body. I saw it as an adversary—an enemy, always failing me just when I needed it most.

I don't know what prompted me to walk into the Tae Kwon Do dojang (training hall) on that June morning. I think I was disgusted with how out-of-control I felt my body had become. And I was out of control in other ways, too. I had little mental discipline and few friends; I had become a very negative, unhappy person. How could I like myself that way—and how could others like me?

The dojang was located near a main street in my town and I drove by it almost every day. I suppose that's why the place felt so familiar to me. When I walked in, I found myself in a tiny waiting room. Beyond I could see an empty training hall. Rows of windows lined the south wall; mirrors and wooden bars were attached to the north and east walls. It reminded me of the school where I had learned ballet as a child, and I suppose this was comforting. Like many people, I had always been curious about the martial arts, but they had always seemed slightly sinister to me. No one I knew participated in the martial arts. I had never thought of trying the martial arts myself, though as a child I had wanted to learn Karate. When

I was a child all martial arts were called either Karate or Kung Fu, without regard to what they really were. I had wanted to learn Karate because I thought it would be great to save someone in distress and to never be afraid of what might happen to me. But like most young girls, I soon quit thinking of myself in the role of a rescuer and instead daydreamed about what *my* rescuer would be like, and when he would arrive. He would resemble a movie star. Maybe he would know Karate.

But now, all these years later, the room I found myself in was reassuring. A small blonde woman wearing a crisp uniform with a black belt asked if she could help me. I said yes—what about signing up for lessons? Could I try a few and see what I thought? I told her I had just quit smoking a few months earlier after emergency surgery to repair one of my lungs, and I wanted to be in better shape. I wanted to lose some weight.

Tae Kwon Do could help with that, she said. She knew what I was really looking for. She knew I was trying to turn myself into a rescuer again, a person who saves others, who saves herself, even, and does not wait for someone else to arrive.

She explained that she and her husband had started the school a few years before. I could see a picture on the wall showing her breaking four concrete blocks with a palm strike. Despite her tiny stature, the room was filled with her presence. There I was, old, fat, out of shape, a short, dumpy brunette, and I wanted to be just like her. And she believed I could be.

I often tell people that Tae Kwon Do saved my life when all I had really expected it to do was help me lose some weight. And that's the reason for this book—that martial arts can change the lives of women. But more practically than that, I wanted to write a book that helped women become better martial artists.

As a martial artist myself, I often try to improve my skills by following the instructions of others, often using videos and books to do so. What I have discovered is a lack of practical advice for female martial artists, if not outright hostility toward us. In fact, I recently saw a martial arts magazine address the topic, "Do Women Belong in Martial Arts?" This is indicative of the nature of most male-oriented martial arts publications. Martial arts books that are targeted toward women tend to be restricted to general self-defense. Female martial artists want and deserve attention to their particular needs and issues. In many ways, female martial artists differ from male martial artists and need information specifically for them. For instance, women are prone to different injuries than men; because of our build, in general, martial arts can be very hard on our hips. Other injuries are also gender-specific, yet little information exists on avoiding them. Since most martial arts instruction is aimed at men, the needs and questions of female martial artists are often overlooked—from how to make the uniform fit better to whether it is safe to practice while pregnant. I have seen plenty of advice on sparring, but what if you are shorter than everyone you spar (as is often the case with women)? I have learned, through trial and error, the value of fighting "inside," but I have always believed that there should be more information on how women can and should spar, capitalizing on their strengths and overcoming their weaknesses. That's what this book is about—providing some of those answers for beginning and advanced martial artists. Most female martial artists should find something of value in these pages.

I must take a moment to thank my instructors, Donald and Susan Booth, without whom I would still be old, fat, out of shape and discouraged; my black belt colleagues, especially those who were gracious enough to talk to me about the material in this book; to my editor, Cynthia Kim, whose kindness and patience has helped me see this project through; to Grandmaster Jung, of Cedar Rapids, Iowa, who started all of this twenty-five years ago, when he arrived in the United States with $35 in his pocket and a dream.

And finally I must thank my husband, Bret Kay, who has seen me on the way with love and laughter, and whose patience has made me a better martial artist.

1

What are Martial Arts?

Martial arts, in the simplest terms, are systems of techniques used for fighting. All martial arts schools emphasize the defensive nature of their training and advocate non-violence whenever possible. The martial arts, however, are not merely collections of self-defense techniques, but are—or should be—holistic approaches to life, stressing harmony and balance between mind and body, between the self and others. They are not religions; if anything, they are philosophies, stressing respect toward others and moderation in all things. Any martial arts school that ignores the philosophy of martial arts is not really a martial arts school at all. It is a fighting school or a self-defense school. While these may be useful, they are also limited in what they can do for you. The best benefits—mental and physical—come from those schools that emphasize the whole mind and body.

The martial arts emphasize the middle way—that is, balance and harmony. The active life should have its contemplative moments; work should be balanced with rest; intensity with relaxation. Martial arts schools also emphasize qualities such as courtesy and dignity as much as they might emphasize power or board-breaking. Most martial arts schools have a formal atmosphere, but once a student is made aware of the rules and expectations, such a structure can be soothing and stress-relieving.

Unlike other sports, martial arts do not rely on or emphasize winning or victory as the only measure of an individual's success. A martial artist can be perfectly well respected by others without ever winning a national title or a street fight, though, of course, there are always people who see such achievements as "proof" of an individual's prowess and worth.

A good martial artist isn't merely technically talented. He or she must also be a good role model, be willing to help others, be a good teacher and be willing to expend as much energy as necessary to improve him or herself. The biggest competition—and the biggest obstacle—martial artists face is themselves. Not only will you compete against others, you will compete against yourself. The martial arts allow you to learn, achieve and grow according to your own speed and abilities. That's why they are so appealing to people of all ages, sizes and physical conditions. No matter where you are now, you can become better—healthier, more fit and less stressed. Older people have successfully trained in the martial arts; there are, in fact, numerous sixty, seventy and even eighty-year-olds who practice the martial arts. Physical disabilities also do not preclude participation. Individuals in wheelchairs can practice martial arts, as can those who suffer from conditions such as cystic fibrosis, multiple sclerosis, and arthritis. Many such individuals have benefitted greatly from their participation in the martial arts.

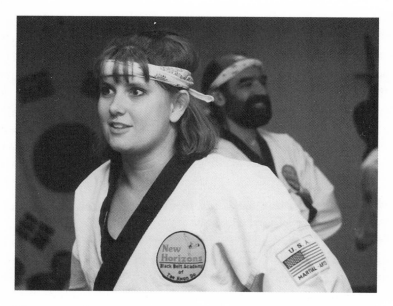

The martial arts are open to men and women of all ages.

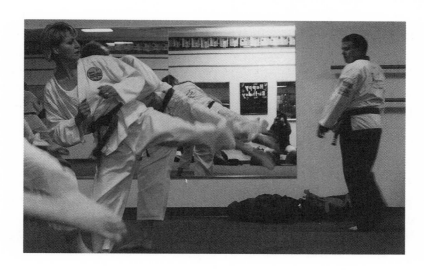

Group training has many benefits.

Though it is possible to train solo, unless you are already very skilled, training solo only will not be rewarding or effective. The martial arts require both individual and team effort. You work hard as an individual to perfect techniques and to learn to control and discipline your mind and body. Yet you don't learn in isolation. You and other students in your school work together as a team. School members work out together, train together, correct each others' mistakes, teach each other and, most importantly, encourage each other. The same individuals against whom you compete in the sparring ring may become your best friends.

Therefore, students are usually very loyal to one another, their school and their instructor. Martial artists are expected to be courteous and helpful to each other and the instructor. They must remember that they always represent their school, whether they are in class or walking down the street. No good martial artist would want to embarrass his or her instructor or cause negative publicity about his or her school. This loyalty has nothing to do with any money you pay to take classes; instead of thinking of martial arts training as a service being purchased, the martial artist must think of training as an agreement. He or she promises to work hard and be loyal to the instructor and school; in exchange, the instructor will help the student become a better martial artist. Of course, prudence dictates that one avoid being taken advantage of, as can happen in any reciprocal relationship.

Martial artists are expected to contribute to the success of their school. This helps the students bond together and ensures dedication and loyalty. This "contribution" is on-going. A martial artist might be asked to give a demonstration of her skills at an open house or to lead a class. Depending on an individual's inclination and abilities, he or she might write a newsletter for the school or vacuum the carpet once or twice a week or something of a similar nature. Like a family, the members of a martial arts school work together to show their pride in themselves, each other and their school.

Teaching is also integral to martial arts practice. All martial artists are expected to help each other learn. Higher ranks (brown and black belts) may be asked to lead class. Students of any rank are expected to assist others and to teach techniques to other students when asked. Teaching is fundamental to learning, according to most martial arts philosophers. The more you teach, the more you must examine your own techniques (and correct them). You must also answer questions; this makes you think about theory and application. Because you are expected to teach, you must always be up to date on all of your techniques so that you can show them with confidence to someone else.

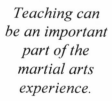

Teaching can be an important part of the martial arts experience.

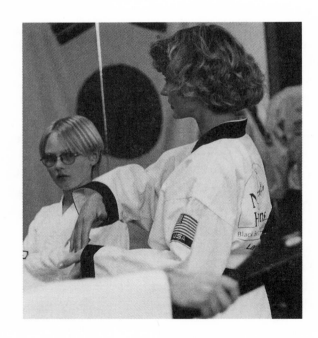

Sport versus Art

Some martial arts styles and schools emphasize the "sport" aspect more than others do. Competing in local, regional and national tournaments appeals to many martial arts practitioners. Such events can be rewarding. They may be stressful, but they help you to see how you respond under pressure. If you routinely perform under pressure, you feel less stress and you respond more effectively.

Some schools, however, are sport-only schools. These schools teach tournament sparring skills and little else. While some people thrive in this environment, most won't. Further, it isn't a true martial arts experience; martial arts aren't simply sports and they certainly aren't just about winning. They are about controlling your mind and body; they are about learning to defend oneself and coming to know who you really are. This holistic approach means that your abilities change as you do—perhaps as you grow older, become more fit, sustain an injury, or otherwise become different. Nonetheless, though your particular circumstances may change, your health and fitness goals can still be achieved. If you are sidelined for a week or two (a sprained ankle or a bad cold), you can still practice some of the elements of martial arts. This keeps you connected so that you will return to training. As anyone who has ever had to be away from a fitness program can tell you, returning is difficult. The martial arts emphasize staying connected, thus making a return much easier.

Martial Arts Skills

Martial arts training varies from style to style, but certain skills are taught by all. Each martial art style has techniques exclusive to that style. For instance, Tae Kwon Do is known for its jumping kicks. These techniques—or the basic versions of them—will be the first thing you learn. Punches, kicks, blocks, take-downs, whatever your particular style emphasizes, you will be drilled in the basic techniques. You will repeat them over and over until you are proficient—and then you will still need to practice every day. These basic techniques, sometimes called basic movements, are essential to the study of martial arts.

Forms, often called *kata* or *hyung*, are also part of martial arts training. A form is simply a set pattern of techniques that a martial artist memorizes and practices. This allows the martial artist to work on techniques in a series and to combine techniques together. Forms emphasize balance and grace; they are the "art" in martial arts. Forms also help build muscles and flexibility. These are usually performed solo, though some styles have partner forms.

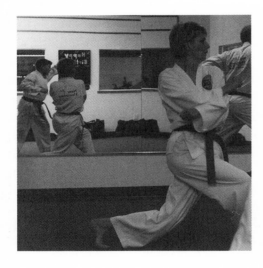

Practicing forms and basic techniques is an important element of most martial arts classes.

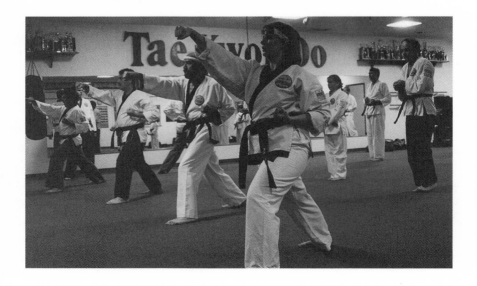

Sparring is the third element of martial arts training. This comes in several kinds. Step sparring is a controlled situation where two partners work together. They have a mock confrontation, with one partner striking and the other responding by blocking and then executing a series of techniques to stop the attacker. When the last movement is concluded, the partners return to the ready position and begin again. Freestyle sparring, on the other hand, allows two partners to fight against each other continuously for a round of several minutes. Both partners attack, defend, and counter swiftly, never stopping (unless score is being kept). Most schools require safety equipment for this. Freestyle sparring is considered to most closely resemble an actual fight situation.

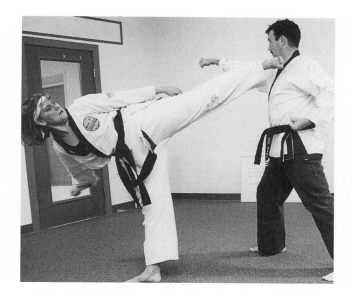

Step Sparring allows controlled practice of realistic skills.

Board breaking is part of the curriculum in some martial arts schools. It is an area of confusion and misunderstanding to many people unfamiliar with the martial arts. Board breaking is integral to some styles, whereas other styles never do it at all. Breaks with the head, which are popular in movies, are never done in reputable martial arts schools; most instructors won't allow it and some will demote students who try. Breaks are done with the foot, the fist, the palm or the elbow. Extremely well-trained martial artists can break boards with their shins, but this is a good way to break a shin instead of a board.

In many Korean styles, students are expected to break boards at each belt level, using more and more sophisticated techniques as they learn more about the martial arts. Such performances have three purposes. The first is to demonstrate power. Obviously, in practice, one cannot kick one's practice partner with full power; this would cause injuries, and sooner or later you would run out of partners. So boards are used instead to demonstrate power, not only to teachers, judges and others, but to the student as well. Breaking a one-inch thick board, the equivalent of a person's rib, can assure the practitioner that he or she can truly defend him or herself. Often it is hard for the practitioner to feel as if he or she could actually generate enough power to ward off an attacker. Therefore, if one can break a board, one can be more assured of possessing the necessary strength and skill for self-defense. The second purpose is to be certain the student is executing proper technique. A board will not break unless the technique used is correctly applied. The final purpose for board breaking is to discipline the mind. It is mentally difficult to actually hit a board. You think, "What if it hurts?" Or, "What if I can't do it?" Overcoming these mental blocks is one of the important points. Board breaking is often more of a mental challenge than a physical one. Schools that don't break boards will have other methods of challenging the mental blocks of the martial artist.

Some schools also teach the use of weapons. Not handguns, of course; they teach things like swordsmanship or staff fighting. These are not necessarily considered practical weapons, but they are practical for the benefits they give; muscle conditioning, quick reflexes, balance, and self-awareness. As anyone who has worked with nunchuks can tell you, weapons training makes you learn coordination quickly. If the idea of learning traditional weapons appeals to you, be certain to ask the head instructor; many schools don't teach weapons. Weapons training can help you get in touch with the essence of the martial arts. Zen training, for instance, always starts with weapons training, at least in traditional schools.

In addition, meditation is often a practice associated with martial arts training. Often, this takes the form of meditation classes which the martial artist is encouraged to attend, but meditation is also taught more informally, through relaxation and visualization exercises that might be conducted as part of the class.

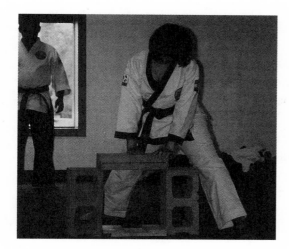

Board or brick breaking is often introduced in advanced classes.

A wide variety of exotic weapons are taught at some schools.

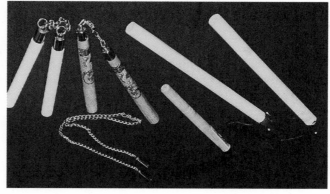

Customs

Ordinarily, students practice or work out in uniforms purchased through the school; many styles require bare feet. This is simply a traditional practice, but wearing a special outfit can help one make the transition from work, school or another activity. Putting on the uniform (sometimes called a "gi" or "dobok") reminds the student that he or she is preparing for martial arts practice. Changing into the uniform focuses the mind on what one hopes to achieve through practice. Usually these uniforms are closed with a belt that indicates the wearer's rank, which is discussed later in this chapter.

At most schools, students are expected to bow to senior belts (those students and instructors who are of higher rank) and sometimes to flags or other symbols. A bow is merely a sign of courtesy, much like a handshake. Such gestures have no religious significance; there is no need to feel uncomfortable about making them. Other forms of etiquette are expected of the martial artist as well. One doesn't interrupt others, for instance, unless the school is on fire. Certain parts of a training workout require complete silence, in deference to the instructor. Elements of courtesy vary from school to school.

Benefits of Martial Arts Training

Martial arts practice develops strength and flexibility for the purpose of self-defense and general fitness. Flexibility is needed to perform many techniques, especially high kicks and jumping kicks in the striking styles; in the grappling styles, good flexibility can help you to pin your opponent and avoid (or escape) being pinned yourself. Such flexibility is also helpful in everyday life; it is one of the benefits of martial arts training. Those with limited mobility will still be able to perform many techniques, and concentrated effort on improving flexibility can help those with limited mobility achieve a greater range of motion.

Strength, of course, is one element of power (speed is the other). Strength is gained through repetition of techniques, though practice of forms and other parts of martial arts training. Many martial artists, however, do eventually begin lifting weights to contribute to their strength, though this isn't necessary. Most new practitioners see a significant increase in strength as well as muscle tone and definition within the first three or four months of training.

The greatest benefit one derives from the martial arts is the focus on developing inner energy. This energy is called "chi" (sometimes spelled "ki" or "qi") Some martial arts practitioners believe chi is life-force and can be controlled and directed against opponents almost magically. Other martial artists, however, simply consider chi to be focused energy. That's why you hear loud yells at martial arts tournaments (or in martial arts movies, just before the hero kicks an attacker). These loud yells (called "kiai" or "kihop" depending on the style) focus the practitioner's energy and attention while he or she performs some powerful move or a difficult technique. Martial artists always kiai before breaking boards and during sparring matches to indicate a scoring attempt. The shout is developed as part of the controlled breathing exercises that are taught in the martial arts. These exercises can be helpful in daily life, for they help to relieve stress or to calm oneself when fearful or angry.

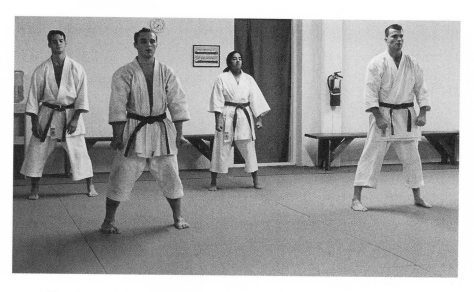

Traditional karate students focus on developing their "chi".

Belt Ranks

All martial arts school expect students to improve with time and training. These improvements are marked by ranks, which are indicated by belt color. Most styles begin with a white belt. The colored belts include yellow, orange, green, blue, purple, brown and red. Not all schools use all colors (some of the colors are interchangeable) and not all colors are ranked in exactly this order at all schools. Black belt is almost always the highest rank a practitioner can achieve. Ranks are sometimes further divided by level; for instance, green belt might have both a "high green" level and a "low green" level, "high" indicating a greater level of competence. This might be shown by a black stripe on the green belt. The black belt itself has various "degrees," usually called "dans." These degrees indicate the length of time one has practiced a martial art, as well as one's skill level. For instance, in Tae Kwon Do, to be eligible to test for the second degree black belt, one must have practiced for at least two years since earning the first degree black belt. The time necessary increases with each degree. As you can imagine, ninth or tenth degree black belts tend to be older folks. In some styles, to earn the higher black belt levels, you must operate your own school or demonstrate that you are actively teaching the art to others, or have somehow contributed significantly to the art.

To move forward through the ranks, which each student is expected to do, formal or informal tests are given at each level. At such a test, a judge (sometimes an instructor from your own school, often an instructor from a different school) will watch you perform rank-appropriate techniques. Students do occasionally fail these tests, but that is usually owing to lack of effort and preparation. Such tests can be valuable, allowing you to learn to perform under pressure and conditions of stress. They also provide good short-term goals for martial arts training.

Rankings are sometimes very important to the beginning martial artist, and while rankings can serve as powerful motivation to do well, they should not be the only thing that motivates you. In no other sport is attitude worth so much. Perseverance is rewarded, not just with physical benefits, but with mental rewards as well. It is a quality all martial artists strive to achieve.

Martial Arts Styles

How you benefit will vary depending on the style of martial art you practice and how much time and effort you are willing to expend. Martial arts styles are divided into hard and soft styles. A hard style, such as Karate, emphasizes blocking, punching and kicking. Such hard styles can help you develop excellent power, good muscle tone and stamina. Hard style training, however, tends to be anaerobic (you end up out of breath a lot). Still, with practice, you can make these workouts effectively increase your lung capacity and improve your overall cardiovascular health. A soft style, such as Aikido, emphasizes using the attacker's own force to off-balance him or her. These styles are especially good for older students and those with physical limitations. A soft style will increase balance, strength and aerobic condition. Each kind of style is equally valuable and worthwhile; the emphasis is merely different. Try to watch artists from both hard and soft styles before deciding which is for you.

Martial arts are also sometimes divided into two different categories—striking styles and grappling styles. Striking styles, such as Tae Kwon Do, emphasize striking or hitting the attacker with fists, feet, elbows and knees. Grappling styles emphasize joint locks (which are extremely painful and can render an attacker harmless) and throws. Judo, for instance, is a grappling style that emphasizes bringing an attacker to the ground. Again, neither kind is necessarily better, but again, one should see the different styles before deciding which to try. Often, success in martial arts is simply a matter of finding the style that suits you best.

The best known styles are also the ones that are most likely to have schools near you. Each style is slightly different. In the United States, the major styles are Aikido, Karate (which has many subcategories, such as Okinawan, Kenpo, etc. All Karate styles emphasize many of the same techniques), Tae Kwon Do, Jujutsu, Kung Fu (also known as Wushu), Judo, and T'ai Chi. T'ai Chi, which some purists do not consider a true martial art, is the gentlest approach to the martial arts and is the most suitable for older individuals, and those with disabilities or other health problems that limit their participation.

There are many other styles of martial arts (including ninjutsu and hapkido) but these styles are less available to the average individual. Because these styles vary, the benefits will vary as well, but each style can contribute to a longer, healthier, saner life.

Aikido

This name means literally "the way of harmony with universal energy." Aikido is a soft style martial art from Japan; it stresses the harmony between mind, body and moral outlook. This purely defensive system was founded by Ueshiba Morihei in 1931, based on the elements of Jujutsu. It emphasizes quick, decisive movements that are designed to turn the attacker's force back on him or herself. This is done through evasive movements and body shifting. An Aikido practitioner does not punch or kick, though he or she may touch the opponent to guide the opponent's body.

The techniques of Aikido are designed to help students to overcome physical and psychological barriers and to become more relaxed and in harmony with themselves and the world around them. Circular movements, without breaks, are used. The circle is seen as a symbol of wholeness and unity which can be used against disharmony, disunity and violence.

The techniques fall into two categories. Certain techniques are designed to control an opponent; that is, the Aikido practitioner will avoid the attack and then move to control the opponent and keep him or her from continuing the attack. The second category consists of techniques designed to throw an opponent. Again, the practitioner blocks or avoids the attack and causes the attacker's momentum to work against him or her. The desired outcome is for the attacker to land on the ground, with the Aikido practitioner in control. Aikido training sometimes includes weapons training; weapons commonly taught are the short, medium and/or long staff.

Karate

Karate means "art of the empty hand." This hard style takes some of its techniques from both Chinese and Japanese martial arts systems. It is a centuries-old art that uses bare hands and feet, though weapons are also part of the training. Karate weapons are usually nunchuks, which have short, baton-like handles linked together with chain; and the tonfa, which consists of a narrow stick with a handle attached to it at a right angle. Such weapons are sometimes used during the performance of traditional forms.

The origins of Karate began when the Chinese occupiers of Okinawa forbade the natives from owning weapons of any kind. Empty-hand fighting was developed by the Okinawan residents to help them defend themselves against troops, thieves, and other rascals. The no-weapons rule is the reason why Karate weapons are so unusual; they are based on farming implements that could double as weapons when needed.

This martial arts system uses striking techniques (kicks, punches, sweeps) to fend off an attacker. No grappling techniques are used (or are necessary). This style is more aggressive than Aikido, which traditionally does not have a sport competition side to it. Karate tournaments are widespread with many participants.

Karate emphasizes powerful blows, speed of movement and timing of attacks. Achieving good, proper technique can take a long time; mastery of the art takes years. This is one of the most widely known and popular styles of martial arts, even though it does require talent and discipline to become proficient. Still, within several months, most practitioners begin to feel comfortable with the basic techniques.

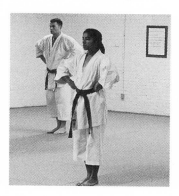

Traditional Karate students practicing breathing exercises.

Tae Kwon Do

Also known as "Korean Karate," the name of this hard striking style means "the art of hand and foot fighting." Like Aikido, this martial arts system was invented within recent memory. The Korean martial arts had become fragmented and disorganized during the Japanese occupation of Korea (from 1910 on), because the teaching of traditional methods of self-defense was banned. Tae Kwon Do was created by a committee of masters in 1955 using elements from older systems of unarmed combat and was named by the Korean General Choi.

Tae Kwon Do, like Karate, emphasizes powerful punches and quick attacks. Tae Kwon Do, however, emphasizes high kicks and jumping kicks that are spectacular and showy, while Karate kicks are focused on the middle and lower parts of the body. The original purpose for this emphasis was to train foot soldiers to kick above their heads; this way they could attack mounted soldiers. Tae Kwon Do has no weapons, nor does it use grappling methods. Sometimes take-down techniques, such as might be found in Aikido, are used. Tae Kwon Do also teaches joint locks and vital point striking. Board breaking, to demonstrate power, technique and mental discipline, is extremely important in this style.

Tae Kwon Do stresses harmony between body, mind and nature. It is only through the correct balance of these three elements that true martial arts achievements can be made.

Judo

"The Way of Gentleness" is a defensive martial art that was created in 1882. This soft grappling style is based on Jujutsu. Judo emphasizes upsetting an opponent's balance, by using her own momentum against her. Like Aikido, Judo techniques include those that control an attacker and those that throw an attacker. However, Judo also relies on a wide variety of grappling techniques, including those used to immobilize an attacker. Joint locking is taught and so are strangulation techniques. Sometimes techniques that can be used against armed attackers are taught. Judo techniques are divided into standing techniques and floor techniques; floor techniques are taught on tatami, or mats. No weapons are taught.

Judo practitioners seek flexibility and balance as well as speed and accuracy of movements. Students are schooled in alertness and mental discipline. The founder, Kano Jigoro, emphasized the philosophy of Judo as a means to a serene and calm mind. With this serene and calm mind, he felt, any attacker could be easily defeated.

Kano Jigoro was opposed to competition from the beginning, since he felt that Judo was a private or personal means of training the mind and body. Judo, however, has become more sport-oriented as the years have passed, and bears more and more resemblance to wrestling than to a true martial art. It has been an Olympic sport for men since 1964 and women's competition was recently added to the Olympic program.

Judo is one of the most popular martial arts in the world, with extremely strong European branches and several million students worldwide. It is an obligatory sport in Japanese schools, and has been since 1956.

Jujutsu

The "science of softness" was created during the twelfth through fourteenth centuries in Japan. This soft grappling style was intended to help disarmed soldiers to fight against still-armed enemies. The basic principle is to defeat the enemy any way possible, using the least amount of force necessary. Like Aikido, Jujutsu emphasizes turning an attacker's own force against him or herself. The opponent is put off balance and immobilized. Jujutsu also emphasizes certain grappling moves and striking to vital areas. The proficient Jujutsu practitioner is expected to be able to gauge the force of an opponent's attack and use that force against the opponent; evade an attack; know how to use leverage against an opponent; and know how to attack without being able to reach weak areas of the opponent's body.

Over the centuries, the basic techniques have been improved upon by many important martial artists. Techniques from Chinese and Okinawan martial arts systems have also been incorporated, which explains why some of the techniques are striking techniques. The methods were actually codified in Japan after the Samurai were no longer permitted to wear swords. This style was first practiced by the Samurai and then by the ninja; after that it became an offensive rather than defensive technique used by thieves.

Early in its history, this ruthless art was feared for its dangerous and often fatal results; modern Jujutsu, however, is less aggressive. Most martial arts derive in some way from this style. Most armed forces teach recruits elements of this close combat style of fighting. Very little sport Jujutsu exists, though this trend is changing.

Kung Fu (Wushu)

More correctly known as "Wushu," the name of this style means "Human Effort." A complete understanding of Kung Fu requires a lifelong effort. Schools vary widely as over four hundred kinds of Kung Fu exist; some kinds of Kung Fu resemble Karate while others resemble T'ai Chi. Therefore, it is difficult to classify it as either a hard or soft style. Grappling methods generally are not used, so it is usually considered a striking style. Weapons are used in some schools, but not all. They vary widely, too, from sword to staff. Kung Fu gained popularity in the sixties and seventies because of Bruce Lee's films and the David Carradine television show, "Kung Fu." In the decades since, it has lost some of it popularity.

All Kung Fu schools teach postures, guards, fist attacks and foot attacks, as well as forms. The schools are classed into Northern styles and Southern styles, with Northern styles being considered those that rely most heavily on foot techniques, while Southern styles are considered those that rely most heavily on hand techniques. In reality, no such distinction can be made between styles.

The distinction that is made is between "inner" and "outer" Kung Fu systems. One emphasizes the "inner" force (chi), vital points and philosophy; the other, "outer", system emphasizes force and rapid movement.

It requires the understanding of Chinese culture, life, history and customs to become truly knowledgeable Kung Fu practitioner.

T'ai Chi

This name means "supreme ultimate fist." T'ai Chi is one of the oldest martial arts in the world; it is so old its origins are lost. Little is known about its early history, though it is credited to the Taoist Chang Zhangfeng. This soft style originated in China. It consists of slow, connected movements that are practiced to reduce tension, to slow breathing, and to clear the mind. T'ai Chi also has weapons, principally a double edged straight sword. Moving correctly and allowing the chi to circulate freely is the goal. Students learn to yield so that the attacker is overcome by his or her own force.

Training consists of three parts. The first part is forms, which are a patterned series of movements. These are done alone. The second part is pushing hands training, which is done with a partner. The third part is weapons forms, which can be done alone or with a partner.

The art emphasizes the middle way, stressing harmony with nature and fellow humans. Students are expected to learn and understand the concept of "yin and yang," or harmony between opposites, a fundamental martial arts principle.

Originally part of the Taoist "Way," this martial art has actually become competitive in some schools, though such competition is contrary to Taoist principles.

T'ai Chi has a stronger spiritual or philosophical side than the other arts described; one direction of T'ai Chi training strengthens bones and muscles while the other direction strengthens spirituality.

2

Attitude

Not long ago, a major martial arts publication ran a feature article titled, "Do Women Belong in the Martial Arts?" The stated concern was that women might not work as hard as men do, or that they couldn't be hit as hard as men could, or that women might distract men (nobody ever points out that this can work both ways). Men, in short, are serious martial artists and women are not. Though the article eventually concluded that yes, men and women can work together without too many difficulties (as long as each and every possible difficulty is anticipated and prudently planned for), the tone was condescending and patronizing, rather like letting your little sister tag along while you and your friends ride your bikes. And that, unfortunately, is an attitude that women encounter all too frequently in the training hall. The fact that the question of women belonging can even be asked indicates that we still have some distance yet to travel. Just remember—and remind others—that whole martial arts systems were founded by women, including Bruce Lee's favorite traditional system, Wing Chun Wushu.

Martial arts, especially in the United States, have long been dominated by young adult men and a few iron women. But more and more, martial arts are attracting practitioners of all shapes, sizes, ages and genders. This benefits everyone, for the rewards of martial art training go far beyond being able to win a street fight or fend off a mugger. There is no reason for martial arts to be limited to only a few especially skilled participants—because most of us, male or female, would not qualify.

The first step toward achieving the greatest benefits from martial arts practice is to find a good martial arts school. For women, the key to a rewarding martial arts experience is to find, specifically, a female-friendly school (see Chapter Nine). By female-friendly, I do not mean easy, watered-down or children's curricula; a female-friendly school is simply one where gender is not an issue and women are as equally welcomed as men. Some women may prefer family-oriented schools, and others may prefer adult-only schools; still others may want a school that specifically caters to women. This is simply individual preference, but all female-friendly schools share certain characteristics, which are discussed later.

Unfortunately, even in the most female-friendly school, women occasionally encounter men who have a condescending or belittling attitude toward them. Because the head instructor sets the tone for the school and is ultimately responsible for all that happens there, if he or she is setting a good example, then such attitudes will be discouraged. For this reason, sometimes the best alternative is to discuss the situation with the head instructor, especially if you are encountering attitudes that might make you quit practicing. Though it may seem petty to report such behavior, rather like tattling to the teacher, it is essential for the head instructor to be aware of any such conduct in his or her school. Negative attitudes cause people to quit, to develop their own negative attitudes and generally sour the entire atmosphere. The head instructor can speak with the offender privately, or perhaps can discuss correct etiquette in general terms with the whole school (a negative attitude is, in fact, poor etiquette). The head instructor can also take special pains to supervise the offending individual more closely, to correct such negative tendencies. But sometimes you might not wish to talk it over with the head instructor and would prefer to handle it yourself.

The first thing you need to decide is how serious the situation is. If you occasionally work with a person who has a cocky attitude, that's just a minor headache, comparable to many minor headaches we deal with each day. Some men refuse to cooperate appropriately. This is especially intimidating if you are at a stage where you need encouragement. Some may even belittle your efforts, or simply stand there and sigh while holding a target that you are attempting to hit. If the person might actually have some useful advice for you or some relevant feedback, try asking for it. If a person is actively involved in your success or failure, he or she will often display a better, more team-oriented attitude.

Such passive, negative behavior is especially difficult to deal with, for the person doesn't commit any overt act to which you can respond. Sometimes ignoring the behavior, and showing it doesn't affect you, makes it disappear. Sometimes it doesn't matter much what you do, you still find yourself in an occasional unpleasant encounter. One of the most important things you can do to minimize the effect such encounters have on you and your martial arts training is to develop a support network of other martial artists, especially other female martial artists. It is important to have the encouragement and support of others as you pursue your martial arts training. Talking, even just in the locker room after class, can help you feel less alone. Women who have been in your situation often have useful advice. Also, if a particular student tends to belittle you, he probably belittles other women as well, and they may have found a successful way of dealing with him. This is true of many situations you may discover in the course of your training. For example, one man I trained with kicked very hard to low target areas, and I was always concerned that he was going to take out my knee. By discussing the situation with others who sparred him, I developed a special strategy for dealing with him, one that I also used in other similar situations. So talking things over with other martial artists can be helpful. Not only can you gain insight, but you'll have people cheering you on and supplying the necessary encouragement to succeed.

As you continue to train, you will develop strategies for dealing with negative attitudes. Often, those students who do have negative attitudes will get to know you and see you as a person, someone who is similar to them. Often this helps them realize how their behavior and attitude toward you should change. Thus, patience, tough as it is, is sometimes your only refuge for dealing with negative attitudes.

Sometimes, however, the situation is a little more serious than lack of encouragement. There are, unfortunately, a number of men (and some women) who think they have something to prove to women, such as they have more testosterone. The delightful thing is when you are a better martial artist than such men and you can beat them in a sparring match, or easily throw them to the mat. However, especially when you are first beginning your martial arts training, such men are sometimes actually superior in skill, though not in personality, and you can't beat them. Sometimes these men can be dangerous, because instead of being passively negative, they are actively negative. Perhaps they spar too hard, or they lack control when they throw you. If this happens, you must immediately speak up and explain that they are being too aggressive and could injure you. In such extreme cases, you should discuss the problem with the head instructor. Among other things, the instructor needs to be aware of such a potential liability, for someone who is overly aggressive with one person is probably overly aggressive with many people. In the worst case, you should refuse to work with a person who lacks proper control and could injure you. This, of course, happens only rarely, and you will probably never encounter a person whose attitude is actually dangerous to you.

Gender Differences

More common is that attitude that is unpleasant because it focuses unnecessary attention on your gender. This is the attitude that many extremely nice men are burdened with. For instance, you might be grappling or sparring, and your uniform top pops open, revealing your sports bra. This happens so frequently as to really not require discussion, but some men will turn bright red and be unable to speak to you for some time after this occurs. Some women wear t-shirts under their uniforms so that when this happens, no one is embarrassed, but my feeling is that men (and women) need to learn to deal with it. A sports bra is not a piece of lingerie. A woman practicing the martial arts is not a sexual object. By not making a big production of gender in the training hall, its importance is minimized.

Other situations that focus men's attention on gender also occur. Perhaps you are sparring with a male partner, and he kicks or punches to your chest, accidentally touching your breast. I have had men stop the match and grovel abjectly for my forgiveness, which is just plain embarrassing for both people involved. If the chest is a target area, of course you are occasionally going to hit a woman's breast. That's simply how it is, but it is very embarrassing for some men, and they make it embarrassing for you, too. With experience, such men quit being embarrassed, so usually your best bet is to ignore it, which also means not drawing attention to any such situations. You might say "no problem" to acknowledge an apology, but don't let it sidetrack you. Sometimes joking can ease the situation, because you acknowledge their embarrassment but also put the incident in its proper perspective. This sort of attention to your gender is more understandable and more forgivable than other kinds of negative attention. Such men are genuinely concerned that they might have hurt you or embarrassed you, so a quick reassurance that this is not the case can help them understand that you aren't the fragile, breakable type.

Sometimes such men, overly concerned with the fact that you are a woman, attempt to encourage or compliment you by saying you are as good as a man. Such comments can be annoying, to say the least, but usually they are meant in a good way. Such men and such comments are just a little misguided. Usually I say "thanks," but I've occasionally been provoked to respond, "and you're as quick as a woman," or "you're as flexible as a child," to help them understand that such comments are not necessarily the best praise you can give. Though we prefer to be judged on our performance, not our gender, such attitudes are easier to handle than are the more misogynistic attitudes.

Unwanted Advances

On occasion, a student may make an unwanted advance. In the family-oriented school where I train, three couples have met and married in the last four years. Obviously, men and women can be attracted to each other even with sweat dripping down their faces. As in any coed situation, it is to be expected, though it often comes as a surprise to women that they also have to deal with unwanted interest in the training hall. If someone makes unwanted advances, and you have turned him down, and he persists, the same rules apply as in other situations. You can complain to the head instructor, you can talk firmly to the offending individual again, you can ask the instructor not to pair you with him in class, you can avoid him by attending different classes from the ones he attends. The least disruptive method, though, is probably to interact with others before and after class, so that he will have less opportunity to bother you. Grab a partner and do partner stretches, for instance. Work on a form with another person. Ignore him while working on improving your skills. This will, in the end, discourage most men. While it is frustrating to encounter unwanted interest in what you might hope to be a neutral environment, it is comparatively rare and can usually be easily managed.

Misconceptions

For the most part, your martial arts experience will be rewarding, but if and when you run into sexist attitudes, try not to let them discourage you. Negativity towards female martial artists is usually the result of misconceptions that men have. Though it is not your responsibility to educate them, unless you want to, an understanding of these misconceptions can help you remain patient. Be aware, however, that in some schools it is acceptable to buy into these misconceptions, to consider women less talented or less important than men. It is imperative to steer clear of such schools. If you are in one now, get out! An atmosphere like this encourages stereotypes, misunderstandings and leads to unpleasant conditions that may easily make you give up on the martial arts. Rest assured that most schools, however, discourage unfair or unequal treatment of women, and it is just a few individual people who may cause you distress.

Misconceptions about female martial artists abound. Non-martial artists think they are unusual, unfeminine and otherwise different from "normal" women. Male martial artists may believe they are not as dedicated, not as talented, not as serious and not as strong. But of course all people are dedicated, talented, serious and strong to varying degrees having nothing to do with gender.

In the martial arts, however, the goal is to create an equal environment, where gender is not a consideration except in extremely limited circumstances (perhaps in women-only classes). In the martial arts the only distinction of any real relevance is that of rank. Therefore it is discourteous not to be respectful to anyone merely because of physical attributes. Some individuals misunderstand the point of martial arts, thinking martial arts are about street fighting, and therefore the weak, the timid and those lacking confidence do not belong. Of course, even if it were true that martial arts teach only street fighting skills, then who better to belong than the weak, the timid and those lacking confidence? People with this attitude, that only certain individuals can and should study the martial arts, tend to be a little cocky and arrogant. They are derisively called "hotdoggers" among my martial arts associates; they probably have other names in other groups, but no true martial artist really thinks that the martial arts are only about street fights.

Most martial artists have never been in a street fight and never will be; in fact, most of us are taught never to use our martial arts training unless we have absolutely no choice. This means you don't pick fights, you walk away from fights, and you do anything *but* fight, unless you are threatened with severe bodily harm. And frankly, very few of us are ever threatened with severe bodily harm. Therefore, the attitudes of such men are ridiculous and are not worth your concern. Even if such a person is quite skillful, remember, nobody starts out as an accomplished martial artist. Learning fighting skills takes time, and in the process you will learn other things as well.

Bullies

In addition to the men who think that martial arts are meant for street fighting and should be reserved only for those who are tough enough, there are sometimes bullies in the martial arts. Bullies and hotdoggers are sometimes the same people, but more frequently, a bully, who picks on children and smaller or less-skilled women, has little self-confidence. He is cowardly and afraid and tries to exert power over others by picking on people who are no threat to him. A bully will never spar too hard with an accomplished black belt, because he might be easily beaten, but he will spar too hard with a young teenager and then attempt to defend his actions by saying that everyone needs to be challenged. Usually bullies grow out of their behavior by adulthood, but if you run into one, he must be met with self-confidence.

Women who are new at martial arts are easily intimidated by bullies, who tend to be overly aggressive, but in this case, you should assert yourself and insist that the person use control. The head instructor should also be consulted, for a bully in the training hall won't be dangerous only to you but to everyone, including himself. But the most important thing to remember is to insist on respect from everyone, including the hotdoggers and bullies in the world. Part of learning martial arts is learning respect, and such people sorely need a lesson in respect! You can and should expect others to be courteous to you and to work at your skill level. It is not wrong for somebody to challenge you to work harder, for this is how a martial artist improves. But there is a difference between helping you to improve and trying to humiliate you.

Respect

Most of the negative attitudes you will encounter have to do with respect, or lack thereof. You cannot force someone to respect you, but you can expect them to be courteous to you. If, for instance, a lower belt is disrespectful, you have every right to point it out. At the same time, you should be certain you are performing necessary courtesies yourself, for sometimes negative attitudes are a result of our own omissions.

It is also important to remember a few points about martial arts. First, most people are expected to teach and to help each other out. You might, therefore, find yourself being instructed quite frequently by people other than the head instructor. This is to be expected. As a student, you should follow the instructions of others, especially of senior belts. It is only if the person's attitude or behavior is inappropriate that you should take action. Some people do not have very good teaching skills, and they might annoy or frustrate you as they give you instructions. But this is one of the things you will learn—how not to show annoyance, how to swallow frustration, and above all, how to be patient. Some people, when assigned to help teach, will be extremely fussy and will criticize everything you do. Try to learn what you can, and vow never to be a teacher like that yourself. In fact, you will be able to learn a lot about teaching from the way others teach you. When it is your turn to teach, try to remember what it feels like to be criticized yourself, and perhaps emphasize what the student is doing well.

Some people who work with you may be confusing, or may seem to contradict something you learned before. Remember, however, that sometimes what we think we were shown and what we actually were shown are two different things. I have discovered this myself as both a student and a teacher. For instance, I have performed a form and the instructor has told me I am doing the wrong technique. I am always positive that I was shown the form that way, and my first thought is that I was shown the form incorrectly. Yet I also know that the people who have taught me forms are extremely competent, so perhaps I merely learned it incorrectly. As a teacher, I have shown students forms, and they will perform them incorrectly, even though I know I have taught them correctly. Thus, the teaching and learning experience requires patience.

If you are uncertain that what you've been taught is correct, ask the head instructor (people do make mistakes). But it would be disrespectful to tell the head instructor, "Joe Smith taught me this form wrong." A better way to ask is to say, "This is how I am doing the form. Is that correct?" The reason it is considered disrespectful to blame someone else for teaching incorrectly is to emphasize the fact that you are responsible for your own learning, and the person who is learning is more likely to make mistakes than the person who is teaching. As usual, learning new forms and techniques is also a lesson in humility.

There is also a difference between disrespect and discipline. For a martial arts school to function, the head instructor must maintain a certain amount of discipline. This is needed for a good learning environment, for the development of character and for the maintenance of safe practice. So you might very well be told to do twenty knuckle pushups because you were looking around during a formal exercise, or because you forgot to bow to a senior belt. This may not seem fair (you may not have known that you aren't supposed to look around during formal exercises) but there is always a reason behind discipline in the training hall. Martial arts classes are not like other classes, so don't expect from your martial arts teacher what you might expect from your dance teacher. The martial arts instructor is also a coach, and must motivate and discipline his or her students as well as teach them. Therefore, if you or the entire class is disciplined for one reason or another, learn what you can from it, but do not take it personally. Of course, it is another matter entirely if an instructor or another student is disrespectful to you, or treats you poorly.

The Right Attitude

The key to successful martial arts practice, however, is not to concern yourself with other people's reactions to you. While a good martial arts school fosters a sense of school spirit, and a sense of community and teamwork, ultimately, you are simply responsible for you. You must focus on giving the martial art your best effort. The less attention you pay to other people's negative attitudes, the less likely such attitudes will affect you, and the less likely such attitudes toward you will continue. Negative behavior or attitudes tend to disappear as the martial artist gains more self-confidence and begins to understand the meaning of the martial arts. Correct practice of the martial arts is, after all, a humbling experience. By this I mean everyone lands awkwardly on the mat sometimes, and everyone finds one opponent who is impossible to throw, and everyone falls down while performing a spinning wheel kick, at least on occasion. It is this reminder of our shared weaknesses that should bond us together as martial artists; it should also help us to develop into better people. In my experience, talented people with poor attitudes do not last long in martial arts training, while less talented people with better attitudes achieve their martial arts goals and continue to practice for years.

And that is the essential element of success in the martial arts— cultivating the right attitude. Sometimes, however, it is difficult to remain positive and confident when others close to you are not supportive.

Balancing Martial Arts and Family Life

Sometimes family members will have difficulty dealing with how much time you spend away from them, practicing the martial arts. Friends, children, spouses and parents all can make it difficult if they don't support you. After all, it takes more time and money to participate in the martial arts than not to participate.

If those around you are not supportive, the best approach to take is to try to educate them. Explain what the martial arts are about and have them visit a class. You may want to tell them of the benefits you receive from martial arts practice. It might make you feel more fit and healthier. Or maybe it helps you feel less stressed. It might give you self-confidence or help you lose weight. Make it clear that these benefits are important to you. Also, setting a schedule and sticking with it helps take some of the pressure off you and your family. If everyone knows that Tuesday and Thursday nights are always Judo nights, they can adjust more easily than if sometimes you are gone on Mondays and Thursdays and sometimes on Tuesdays, Fridays and Saturday mornings, or what have you. Setting a schedule helps others cooperate as well. If your husband knows you always work out on Mondays and Wednesdays, and that it is his job to feed the kids, chances are the entire operation will run more smoothly than if no one, including you, knows when you plan to practice this week. In my case, I had a group of friends who didn't really understand my attachment to the martial arts. All they knew was that brown and black belt class was on Fridays, and that I always went. This meant that if they wanted to get together with me over the weekend, it needed to be Saturday night. It was simply not negotiable, and soon no one really paid attention, they simply remembered to schedule events for Saturday nights.

For your family, more drastic measures may have to be taken. You may need—or simply want—to get them involved. Just as having a workout partner helps you go to the gym three times a week, having another member of your family practicing the martial arts with you can help you both stay motivated, even during those times when you are frustrated with your progress. Spouses who work out together can encourage each other and support each other; your spouse can at least give it a try to find out why you devote time and money to it. Children, if they are old enough, are also often interested in the martial arts. You may wish to sign them up for a few lessons either at your school or another school. If they are involved, too, they will be much more tolerant of the time you spend at martial arts practice. Just as spouses who work out together stay involved in the martial arts longer, so too do families who work out together stay involved. In the past few years, I have seen at least five father-son combinations reach black belt level together, as well as one mother-daughter combination and an entire family. Other such combinations of family members are at various levels of their training now.

If you are younger or single, your parents can also present difficulties. My own parents and siblings thought what I was doing was slightly sinister, so I began inviting my parents to promotion tests (which are, in most schools, open to the public). For my black belt test, I invited my brother and sisters, who brought their spouses and children, as well as my parents. Everyone was quite fascinated; some understood what the martial arts were about better than others, but now everyone has a more realistic idea of what I do.

For other people, friends are not supportive. Again, this is more commonly a frustration among young, single people who rely on their friends for approval and encouragement. Frequently, people have only been exposed to martial arts as practiced by Bruce Lee, Steven Seagal or Jean-Claude Van Damme. They realize that true martial arts practice is not like this, but how it is different, they do not know. Thus, their misconceptions are at the root of any teasing or lack of understanding that you may encounter. When this is the case, providing further information can help. Good friends will eventually understand. This doesn't mean that the friends who continue to tease you should immediately be dumped and never spoken to again, but you will have to refrain from talking about martial arts around them to avoid giving them the opportunity to make comments or sarcastic remarks. If they still do, ignore the comments. Often, friends also just need to be told about the benefits of the martial arts—things like self-discipline, fitness and health.

Sometimes you can express your own misgivings about the martial arts, which also helps your non-martial artists friends to appreciate what you are doing. When I was a yellow belt, a very beginner, I watched a black belt test for his second dan (degree). Part of his test required that he break a concrete block with a punch. He failed on the first try, but managed to open a gash on his hand that bled everywhere. Then he had to try to break the block again, which he did. But I seriously contemplated never testing for my second dan, should I ever attain the rank of black belt.

I immediately went home and called a friend who thought what I was doing was weird anyway. I told her this story, which gave her a little respect for the person who could still hit a block with a bleeding hand, but I also told her my misgivings, which reassured her that I was not crazy. Then we laughed and decided that to ever attain black belt, you must have to lose a lot of brain cells, including those that have anything to do with common sense. Such discussions helped her understand the challenges I faced and while she never was interested in the martial arts herself, she began to understand why I was fascinated. From then on she was always curious about how classes were going and what I had learned. Letting your friends in on your doubts and insecurities as well as your triumphs and rewards helps them put the whole martial arts adventure into perspective, and might even motivate them to participate as well.

But whether your friends and family support you or not, and regardless of any attitudes you might encounter in the training hall, it is the matter of your own attitude that counts. With the right attitude, you can become a better martial artist than you ever imagined. Cultivating a winning spirit is necessary to the martial arts.

Intrinsic Motivation

Winning spirit is not about winning exactly but about becoming a better martial artist and in consequence a better person. The basic ingredient here is to worry about your own conduct, not about what others do. By focusing on developing your own skills, you avoid the poisonous effects of comparing yourself with others and subsequently criticizing yourself—or others—inappropriately. This is not to say that you should not evaluate others as models and attempt to emulate or imitate people who are better than you, because that is one of the ways martial arts skills are taught. But it would be wrong to sell yourself short because of a comparison.

If your instructor is eighteen, slender and extremely flexible, and you are forty-five, have had three children, and can't touch your toes, this doesn't mean you can't be an excellent martial artist. It merely means that you can't be an eighteen-year-old, slender and extremely flexible martial artist. It may mean that you have to work on gaining flexibility, but it mostly means that you will have to achieve your goals in a different way. Perhaps the eighteen year old is extremely quick. Well, maybe you can be powerful. Too often, when we compare ourselves to others, we either sell ourselves short (I'll never be eighteen again, so I'll never be a good martial artist) or we give ourselves excuses (I'll never be eighteen again so I'll never be flexible).

You may have to work harder than a young kid to develop speed, and you may have to work harder than a man to develop power, but you can capitalize on your strengths and be better than both if you put your mind to it. Physical disabilities are not necessarily a limitation either. Certain conditions will require adaptation; for instance, someone in a wheelchair will focus on techniques that can be done with the hands and arms, but such a person can also become a skilled martial artist. At my school, one student has muscular dystrophy and has less control over his muscles and motor skills than anyone else, but he has developed better control than he has ever had before, plus he has developed a self-confidence and self-esteem that are the result of the intense effort of trying to become the best martial artist possible. I happen to have rheumatoid arthritis which affects all my joints, but I can still kick high above my head and can do full splits in all directions. Not that such flexibility was by any means easy to attain or pain free; I was also at the disadvantage of starting martial arts practice when I was in my late twenties. But I was never allowed to use either of these conditions as an excuse for not doing my best, so I overcame some drawbacks to become a better martial artist than if I had been easier on myself.

When we compare ourselves with others, often we shortchange them as well. We think their techniques are sloppy or they demonstrate very little power. This may be true, but it is a poor attitude to take. It is not a good idea to say, "I'm better than he is, because his techniques are sloppy." This benefits no one. You can acknowledge that perhaps another person needs work, but look at yourself first; we can all improve. Unless you are helping instruct another person to improve, it is really not your concern to judge them. By remaining less judgmental than perhaps we are tempted, we develop our own characters. Even if you do find yourself in the position to teach someone who is not as good as you are, you must keep your ego out of it, and find good things to say as well. In the martial arts, a true winning spirit is built on your continual attempt to do your best and then to do better than that. It has nothing to do with how others around you look.

One of the most important elements of doing your best is developing enough self-confidence to trust yourself. Frequently, women enter the martial arts with little experience in other sports. They are not as comfortable with their bodies as conditioned athletes are, and so they are afraid of either hurting themselves or someone else. The physical contact of the martial arts can be a frightening thing, especially when you hear people in the locker room joking about their injuries. Women new to sports are also not accustomed to physical contact; men, even if they did not play organized sports, are more likely to have played rough-and-tumble football games or to have gotten into fist fights and the like. Comparatively speaking, few women have been in fist fights or played tackle football, especially as adults. Bumps and bruises do come with the territory— martial arts practice is not step aerobics or ballet. But the initial difficulties with physical contact can be overcome by cultivating the right attitude.

Being in the proper frame of mind, and trying to appear confident, not fearful, can be helpful. So can such simple things as warming up, which will help your *body* get into the proper frame of mind, as it were. This reduces the chance of a strain or pull, and it also helps improve flexibility and muscle control, which are important in martial arts practice. But the most important way to overcome reluctance to hit or be hit is to practice. You can practice hitting a heavy bag, or you can shadow box until you feel more relaxed. Try to hit the heavy bag using different amounts of force so that you can hit it lightly when you want and you can hit it powerfully when you want. Practice falling to the ground. If you practice a grappling art, such as Judo, the first thing you will learn are ukemi, or breakfalls. It is essential to master these through continued practice.

Winning Spirit

The confidence that develops as a result of such simple physical practice will help you to cultivate a winning spirit. If you are not afraid of accidentally hurting someone or getting hurt yourself, you can apply yourself more completely to the practice of martial arts.

Other qualities are necessary to winning spirit as well. In Tae Kwon Do, the ultimate aim of practice is the development of five qualities that make up a good person. These tenets of Tae Kwon Do are courtesy, integrity, perseverance, self-control and indomitable spirit. Taken together, these five qualities are the essence of true winning spirit. Courtesy helps to create an environment where ego is not supreme. Integrity governs all dealings with others, which we must always conduct honestly. Perseverance helps prevent us from giving up, even when a challenge or task seems impossible. Self-control has to do with both physical control of the body and mental control of the emotions, so that we are restrained physically and emotionally, using reason and judgment, not fear or anger, to make our decisions. Indomitable spirit is having the right attitude whether we win or lose. These qualities, of course, apply to our personal lives as well as our martial arts practice. In Tae Kwon Do, the instructor will sometimes choose to test one or more of these qualities, perhaps by asking you to do something you have never done before. Your cheerful attitude shows your indomitable spirit. Or perhaps you cannot remember all the movements in your form. The instructor, instead of telling you, may merely watch as you struggle to remember. Your ability to not give up and to arrive at the right answer is a sign of perseverance.

When your instructor talks about such guidelines for your conduct, be certain you listen carefully and take him or her seriously. Each style of martial art may ask you to cultivate different qualities, but essentially all such qualities help to develop winning spirit and good character.

Sometimes a school focuses on the cultivation of chi (sometimes called ki or qi). Chi is simply the life force or vital energy inherent in all things in the universe. It is thought that chi is located in the abdomen, where it is controlled through breathing. This essential energy, which unites all things, is creative and active. Martial artists attempt to summon it through the use of the shout or kiai (also known as a kihop). Correct use of chi, it is thought, can make a person more powerful than physical strength alone. The Japanese believe that chi can be detected in one's personality. Therefore, a strong chi is reflected in a strong personality.

Chi, for most American martial artists, is less mystical and is more closely identified with the ability to focus all one's energy and determination on a single target or a single task. In some ways, then, development of chi is important to the development of a winning spirit.

Another quality important to a winning spirit is what the Japanese call fudoshin, which is the ability to remain calm and detached when confronted with a threat or a difficulty. This principle was developed by the famous Japanese warrior-philosopher, Miyamoto Musashi, whose *Book of Five Rings* is essential reading for all martial artists. By remaining calm and detached, one is less concerned about physical harm. This reduces fear and confusion. The person who learns fudoshin can react to a threat or a difficulty with a clear, open mind, and is thus better able to formulate an acceptable strategy than one who panics or merely reacts blindly. Fudoshin, then, is part of self-control. You must have fudoshin to create heijo-shin, another important quality for the martial artist. Heijo-shin is an intensely focused mind, which you must have before any great test. A person who has heijo-shin is relaxed and confident, but focused and determined. Some martial artists say they can see when another person has heijo-shin. Fudoshin and heijo-shin help you remain alert and ready, which reduces fear, surprise and confusion.

Such states of mind are crucial for tests of any kind, both literal and figurative. They are developed through meditation and through physical exercise. But such mental attitudes are nothing without heart or spirit. A martial artist can possess great technical skill and can even have fudoshin, but if she does not also have kokoro, which is heart or spirit, she will ultimately fail. A martial artist without heart or spirit is not a true martial artist. Many times the person with kokoro, who may otherwise possess inferior technical skill, can defeat one who has great technical skill but no heart. Ultimately these qualities derive from the conviction that you are doing your best.

According to the Japanese, five rules should govern the behavior of all athletes, martial artists in particular. These are practical concepts that help the martial artist develop winning spirit. First, you should believe in the philosophy of your school. Secondly, you should stay fit regardless of circumstances (time, money, etc.). Also, you must be committed to mastering martial art skills once such a study is undertaken. In addition, the martial artist must be willing to participate in difficult training. Finally, the martial artist must do her best in competition. These elements, called "Resolute in Five Respects," are thought to be fundamental to successful martial arts training. Essentially, one cannot give excuses for not trying hard and doing one's best.

Funakoshi Gichin, the founder of modern Karate, modified these rules slightly and developed five regulations to which he insisted on strict adherence. These include the necessity for being serious about training, to avoid ego, to be self-aware, to concern oneself with training, not theory, since studying theory gave one the excuse to quit training, and finally to be ethically responsible in all areas of life. Being committed to these rules, Funakoshi thought, would help the student develop a winning attitude.

Equally important are the qualities that must be avoided to develop a winning attitude. Fear, doubt, surprise and confusion all work to defeat the martial artist, and all stem from the martial artist's attitude. Through continual practice of the martial arts, one can learn to control these destructive qualities and encourage the development of more constructive qualities.

The final necessary element in developing a winning spirit is an understanding of yin-yang (variously called ura-omote, in-yo, am-duong, um-yang and cuong nhu tong thoi). This term expresses a concept of the universe as consisting of conflicting but harmonious elements that depend on each other for their meaning. For example, night and day have no meaning except in relation to each other.

Yin is symbolic of the negative, destructive force of the universe, characterized as passive and feminine. Yang is symbolic of the positive, creative force of the universe, characterized as active and masculine. Thus, the opposites combine to make a whole. The martial artist must combine the hard and the soft, the passive and the active, to achieve complete mastery of the art. Yin-yang is a concept that underlies all martial arts and much Eastern philosophy. Martial artists who understand yin-yang also practice moderation in all things.

Developing a winning attitude is based on having heart, refusing to become discouraged, and giving the best effort possible. With this attitude, the marital artist can achieve beyond her expectations and continue to grow in understanding herself and the martial arts.

3

Practical Advice

Women in training have some specific concerns. There are injuries, pregnancy and childbirth. There's menstruation, and menopause, tough at any time, especially hard when you're trying to become a better martial artist. Some women breeze through those times of the month with no problem, get through menopause all right and wonder what the rest of us are talking about. This chapter is not for them; it is for the rest of us.

Other women, who have been active most of their lives, have developed methods for handling these concerns. For those of us who are in neither category, advice from the experienced can help.

First, there's no reason not to exercise during menstruation or menopause. In menopause, hormone levels vary, so one's energy level varies. One is more sensitive to climate and can suffer hot flashes and experience vascular (migraine-like) headaches. Exercise can help ease these conditions. It also helps maintain strong bones and muscles, so that these don't deteriorate during and after menopause, as often occurs. You may be more prone to injury during and after menopause than you were before. Thus, it is especially important to prevent injury. In addition, good stretching can help you maintain flexibility, which many women complain is their first physical ability to go. Continuing martial arts training—even starting martial arts training—will keep you strong and flexible physically and mentally throughout the rest of your life. Certain martial arts are gentler and cause fewer injuries. Yoga, which is not strictly a martial art, incorporates many martial arts components and is a good choice for older women who wish to remain fit but do not wish to take on the challenges of spinning heel kicks. Many forms of Wushu, (known as Kung Fu by Westerners) also appeal to older women who may wish to work on self-defense techniques but who may not be into lifting weights. T'ai Chi is also ideal for older women who want to remain vigorous and mobile without sparring.

Menstruation

For those of us who menstruate on a regular basis, simple problems occur. With all that kicking and stretching, it is easy to leak. This sometimes causes women to avoid training during their period, which is not a good solution at all. First, remind yourself that no one cares. Adults should be able to handle it, kids ignore it, only you are worried about it. But some women will use two forms of protection to help keep this from happening. Some women, especially those with stress incontinence from childbearing, wear disposable absorbent undergarments. These are perfect for women whose menstrual periods are heavy. They are, indeed, cumbersome, and may seem to restrict movement slightly, but they are a much better solution than not working out at all. Since all martial arts styles insist on practicing in very loose clothing, no one will notice. If you feel self-conscious, get a uniform in the next size larger. Or, some martial arts allow dark outfits to be worn (especially among the higher ranking belts.) Check out this option to make you feel more comfortable. I've worn biker shorts under my uniform if I think I might leak. Since my hip injury, I wear compression shorts anyway, so this gives me additional confidence. Something like this may be all that is necessary for you. Biker shorts and the like can be easily found in the women's athletic wear department of most bigger clothing stores.

Since the menstrual cycle occasionally causes bloating and tenderness, you may want to keep a looser fitting practice outfit around for those days. You may feel tired, sluggish and weak; while this can't be overcome, instead of becoming frustrated, redirect your martial arts goals. Work on stretching more during those times when you feel as if your speed is lacking. Practice forms if you can't bear the thought of bag kicking.

Drink plenty of water before class when working out during your cycle. You'll probably become fatigued more quickly and easily than usual. Good nutrition can help. Your doctor can advise you on using supplemental iron tablets if this seems indicated. The reason for fatigue during menstruation has to do with having less blood and less iron in your blood than usual.

Although you may be tempted to take painkillers for menstrual cramps, keep in mind that some painkillers may prevent you from realizing you have injured yourself. Some medications, including anti-inflammatories, commonly prescribed for swelling, can cause stomach upset, abdominal cramps and the like. If these symptoms suddenly appear while you're working out, you could have a problem. Such medications can also cause dizziness, which will interfere with your balance and with your ability to respond quickly. This rules sparring out; other kinds of martial arts practice could be slightly dangerous, so be careful. Those medications that say "Don't operate heavy equipment" should also say, "Lessens your ability to respond to a kick in the martial arts classroom." Ask your doctor or pharmacist about these and other possible side effects.

Don't eat just before you workout. The digestive process will make you even more sluggish and you might upset your stomach. But an empty stomach, combined with menstruation, can feel awful, so try this instead: eat small snacks throughout the day. Eat a small snack, nothing more substantial than an apple, about an hour before you plan to work out. Drink several glasses of water—fill up on fluids—during the hour before class. Try a sports drink with extra carbohydrates in addition to water. Some people chew a Tums or other tablet for indigestion to get rid of excess stomach acid. Stop the liquids about twenty minutes before class. This gives you time to go to the bathroom, as you will certainly need to. Drinking at least 16 ounces and preferably 24 ounces of water before working out will keep your stomach full, without diverting energy to digestion. A sports drink will give your body carbohydrates to fuel your workout, as will an apple or other small snack. This will help you to feel less tired and more energetic. Again, consulting with your martial arts associates can also provide valuable help.

Dressing for Class

In addition to these discomforts, one of the first things a female martial artist discovers is that most everything—from practice uniform to headgear—is actually made to fit men. This doesn't mean that there aren't good pieces of equipment for women—just that they aren't obvious. It requires some patience to find the things you need.

The first thing to remember is that unless otherwise specified, all equipment and uniforms are in men's sizes. Also, for small women, remember that larger children's sizes may fit. All doboks (uniforms) by a company, for instance, will be made the same way, just smaller or larger. This means that for women, regardless of whether they purchase an adult size or a child size, the uniform will fit strangely. Uniform tops button or wrap on the opposite side, left over right, instead of our usual right over left. All pants are cut with waist and hips of relatively similar proportion. Thus, if you get pants to fit your hips, the waist will be huge. If you get pants that fit your waist, they will pull up no further than the middle of your thighs.   Tops don't have darts. If your chest size is medium or larger, and you get something to fit across your bust line, it will be too long and the sleeves will hang past your fingertips. For these problems, a seamstress can help. Also, an entrepreneur could seize the opportunity and start making women's sizes. If you are handy with a needle, you can handle the simple revisions that make the uniform more comfortable.

All uniforms should fit loosely, allowing for comfortable movement in all ranges. But you shouldn't have to worry about your pants sliding down, or your top gaping open. Simple darts in the top will improve the fit. For sleeves that are too long, simply roll them up and stitch a few stitches to keep them in place. If this is not allowed at your school (it does look pretty casual), hem the sleeves. Additional snaps or velcro closures on tops will help them stay securely closed as you work out. Many women simply wear high neck or turtle neck t-shirts beneath the uniform top to prevent overexposure. For pants, darts at the back can improve fit. Also, elastic waistbands are preferable to the drawstring type for many women (you can't get the drawstring type pulled tightly enough around the waist—too much material bunches up. This also makes the pants uncomfortable to wear.) If the elasticized pants have a waist that is too big, replace the elastic with a smaller length of a tighter weave. Hem up pants that are too long. Some women like to buy a few uniforms at a time and fix them all at once.

Don't wear makeup. It runs, smears on the uniform, and otherwise looks foolish. Mascara will get into your eyes and foundation will drip onto your uniform making a stain that is very difficult to remove. Nails should always be trimmed, fingernails and toenails both. Toenails should be clipped back considerably and kept filed; many martial arts are practiced in bare feet and nothing is worse than getting cut by your partner's toenail. They can feel like razors! Likewise, keep your fingernails short. Artificial nails of any kind can be quite dangerous, especially if they catch on loose clothing. They may not immediately break but instead pull and injure your fingers. Also, long fingernails can be dangerous for your partners. Long polished nails are out of place in the martial arts training hall. Among other things, you can't even make a fist correctly! Keep your nails trimmed and filed at all times.

Your hair is also a concern. If it gets in the way as you practice, consider a shorter cut or keep it pulled back. Hair in your face makes it difficult for you to see what you're doing. If you don't want to pull it back in a pony tail because that causes breakage, consider a loose braid. This keeps hair out of your face, and since it is loosely braided, causes less damage to your hair. To keep sweat out of your eyes—and if you have lots of hair, your scalp will sweat more, so you'll have lots of sweat— try tying a rolled up bandanna around your forehead. This absorbs perspiration, looks okay (martial artists get to wear headbands if they want) and also helps to keep your hair out of your eyes.

To find any special clothing or equipment you might need, *The Black Book: The Quarterly Martial Arts Supplies Guide and Master's Desk Reference* is a good place to start looking for anything related to martial arts. Century Martial Art Supply and Kwon, Inc are two of the larger companies who sell martial arts equipment for women. Ask your instructor for any catalogs he or she may have; many supply houses, though they don't so advertise, have women's equipment in stock. There are groin guards and chest protectors for women. Some of the chest protectors are worn under the uniform. Headgear with face protectors are a good choice to keep your nose from getting broken.

Now that it is no longer unusual to see women practicing the martial arts, more is available to them. But it is still not unusual for only a few women to belong to a school, or for a woman to be the only woman in a class. The National Women's Martial Arts Federation can help you feel less isolated. They hold training camps and seminars. Contact: Special Training, NWMAF, P.O. Box 820, Kings Park, NY 11754.

Clothing Sizes

Most karate-type uniforms are sold in a strange set of sizes—000 to 7, 000 being for the smallest children, and 7 being for the biggest men (both height and weight are taken into account when measuring for martial arts uniforms). Women who wear petite sizes, and who are size eight and under will fit into a three; women up to about 5'6" and 170 can wear a four; taller and heavier women will find a five a better choice.

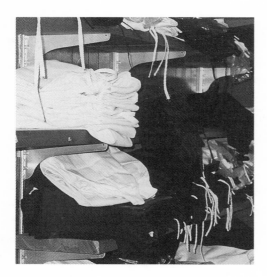

A visit to your local martial arts supply house will reveal a wide variety of uniform choices.

Other martial arts clothing is sold in men's sizes. Having an idea of how men's sizes compare with women's sizes can be helpful. A small men's is like a medium women's. A medium is like a large and a large is like an extra large. That is, men's sizes run a size larger than the same size in women's wear. Men's pants may be sold in traditional sizes, such as 32 x 34. The first number indicates the waist size in inches, and the second indicates the length or inseam size in inches. A 32 x 34 is therefore a pair of pants with a 32 inch waist and a 34 inch inseam (or length). Pant sizes are difficult for women to judge since their hips are usually much larger than their waists, so going by waist size may not yield the correct fit. For an average 5'5" woman who wears a size 12, a men's 32 x 30 is about right. Minor adjustments, such as hemming, may be needed. A 34 x 32 pant would fit a size 14 or 16 woman who is taller - 5'7" or so. Men's clothes usually go up in one-inch increments—the next size up from 34 x 32 is 35 x 32, but sometimes only the even numbers are sold, so the size up from 34 x 32 in a certain piece of clothing might be 36 x 32. This means that you will probably find that you need to make some adjustments. Pants may also be sold small, medium and large; there is usually a one size difference between men's and women's clothing when it is sold like this—a man's large is like a woman's extra-large.

Casual-type clothes, such as men's pull-over shirts, are often sold small, medium and large. Because of the bust line, however, women may feel more comfortable in men's clothing that is slightly larger than what they would wear in women's clothing. I'm most comfortable in loose tops, so while I take a large in women's clothes, I also wear a large in men's clothes. This assures me the looser fit that I prefer. Men's clothes, especially anything fitted, that buttons, snaps or wraps, has much less ease in the chest area than comparable women's clothing. In shirts that are sized conventionally, by collar size, keep in mind that again there is less ease in men's clothing than in women's. A 17 or 17 ½ collar size would fit a size 14 woman though it will be loose. A woman of this size would probably be comfortable in size 16 - 17 ½, depending on how closely-fitting she prefers her clothes. A size 12 woman might be comfortable in the 15 - 16 range. Sometimes a chest size is also indicated on men's clothing. For instance, a size 17 ½ collar might also indicate that it is for a size 36 chest. This is helpful in determining the appropriate size. A 36C bust measurement would work in this size shirt. A half size smaller, say a 17 collar, 35 ½ chest, might work for a 36A or 36B woman. Again, it may take some experimentation, but especially when ordering through the mail, it helps to have an approximate idea of the size you'll need.

For sparring equipment, keep in mind that men's sizes are about one size larger. Small gloves will fit a woman with medium-sized hands. For footgear, usually sold in small, medium and large sizes, it's helpful to know that a medium would fit a woman's foot size 8 to 9 ½ or 10. Large fits size 10 and above. Small works for size 6 and 7. If you wear a smaller shoe size and an extra small is not available, try some of the larger children's shoe sizes. Martial arts shoes and sometimes footgear might also be sold by regular men's sizes. Men's 3 - 13 is the usual range. Men's shoes are about a size and a half larger than women's. A woman who wears a size 9 show will probably be comfortable in a men's size 7 ½ or 8. Again, foot width as well as length and personal comfort will affect the actual size that works best, but these measurements should give you an idea of where to begin. Once you are familiar with the differences between men's and women's clothing and men's and women's sizes, you may choose more specifically what will work for you.

Keep in mind that tunic-type tops and elastic waistband or drawstring pants offer the most flexibility for female martial artists. They require the least number of adjustments and tampering. Again, always be open to discussing these questions and concerns with other martial artists. Even if there are few women at your school, there's a whole martial arts community out there—and it's usually a good one, worth belonging to.

Kihop

In the attitude chapter, I discussed ways to handle the sort of gender-related stereotypes that you might come across. One of the consequences of this is that you become the standard by which other women are judged—which can be a bit of a burden, if you think about it. As a female martial artist, it's important to be a good role model for other women and girls, too. This can work in surprising and unexpected ways. I've seen men ask my husband pointers on a special jump spinning heel kick he does; no one asks me about my jump reverse kick even though it's extremely powerful. What they do ask me about is my kihop—also called kiop or kiai, or shout.

Many martial arts cultivate the use of the kiai (from chi or ki, which is like life energy) as a way to focus and generate power and force. One lower belt mentioned that she had modeled her kihop after mine (although all the black belts tease me mercilessly about it, claiming they can hear it when they're at home and I'm at class). It had never occurred to me that someone would consider my shout worthy of emulating. Another time a younger woman approached me and said, "Your kihop cracks me up," and then added seriously, "Just how do you do it?" I showed her how to yell from the solar plexus, not the lungs, and she immediately felt the difference. Women tend to have more soprano voices and their yells can be thin and breathy. Men naturally have slightly lower yells, so even if they're doing it incorrectly, it often sounds okay. And some people (usually kids) just scream, which is not the effect that anyone is looking for.

If your kihop needs some work, try letting out a long yell. Feel where your breath comes from. Most of the time it comes from your upper chest or diaphragm. Then, repeat the yell, this time putting your fist on your solar plexus. As you yell, push on your solar plexus. You'll immediately hear a change in the tenor and tone of your shout. This can be encouraging because the shout may make you feel more powerful. It can help you focus your energy, thereby helping you to improve your martial arts performance. It can also make you feel more confident.

The shout can also be difficult because women aren't used to doing so—yelling, drawing attention to themselves. This is where your experience is a cheerleader will help. For those of us who were never cheerleaders, the yell may make you feel foolish. But remember, all of the other students are focused on themselves, and how foolish they feel. Other people are always more worried about what they themselves are doing than what you are doing. You'll realize after a while that you don't even notice other people's yells; therefore, why would they notice yours? Being self-conscious makes the whole process more difficult. Remember, everyone else has been in your shoes, feeling awkward. It is actually a lot of fun to yell, and after a while it becomes such a habit that you don't realize that you are doing it—until someone draws your attention to it, like my two students did.

Perseverance

Developing the confidence to yell loudly without inhibition can be fun and rewarding. It can also help you learn to do your techniques with confidence. Doing techniques well requires the right speed, timing and power—none of which you'll have if you're tentative or unsure. I always encourage people to make a commitment to the technique—even if you do end up executing it incorrectly. I'd rather see an incorrectly performed low block done with enthusiasm than a perfectly done low block performed slowly with little confidence. Even if the enthusiastic low block isn't perfect, it has a much better chance of being successful and doing what it is supposed to do (i.e., block the low section from attack) than a block correctly done with little interest or effort.

Because Tae Kwon Do relies heavily on kicks, much of the time is spent learning how to jump in the air, spin, and balance on one foot. As you might imagine, people fall down while doing this. At first, lower belts are very embarrassed if they fall down while practicing a kick. But, at my school, we always say (and mean) "If you're not falling down a lot, you're not trying hard enough." If you commit to your techniques so much that you sometimes fall down trying to kick higher, faster or stronger, you're on the right track. If you never make such mistakes, you are either so vastly talented that this book is completely unnecessary to you, or you aren't trying hard enough. While you want to reach perfection even in practice, you should also be unwilling to settle for what is simply comfortable. It isn't practice that makes perfect, but perfect practice that makes perfect, as so many sports philosophers have pointed out. But unless you are constantly attempting to outdo and challenge yourself, you aren't practicing perfectly. The martial arts are the one place where you can try and fail and try and fail and no one even notices the failing—just the trying.

Women, especially those who have not been athletic in the past, do bring more self-consciousness to martial arts than men do. They are also much harder on themselves than men are, wanting to do things correctly, right away, immediately. This can be frustrating. It can also be discouraging. Just remember the martial arts are about you becoming better than you were—and it takes time and effort for that to happen.

A good martial artist isn't necessarily one with an awesome roundhouse kick. It might be someone how can coach amazingly, so that others who wouldn't believe it possible can do awesome roundhouse kicks. Every person finds her place in the martial arts, maybe as the superstar who impresses everyone, or maybe as the one who perseveres and inspires others to follow suit. I certainly never thought I'd be the kihop lady—I'd sure like people to be impressed with my jump reverse kick—but my kihop is my very own—it's my little corner of the martial arts world, it's one thing I am very good at, and it's something other martial artists always notice about me.

Martial arts are about growing and becoming more fit, more flexible, and stress free. This only works when you release your self-criticism and enjoy what you can do and what you do well. This doesn't mean we should not be critical of ourselves or that we don't need to strive for improvement. It simply means we should give ourselves a chance and not write ourselves off too early in the game.

Adjusting to Contact

Because many women who take up martial arts have not been athletic, they have other concerns as well. Even among athletic women, most are used to non-contact sports, such as tennis, biking, and track and field. Those who work out to keep fit might take aerobics classes, lift weights, walk the treadmill and the like. Sometimes they are used to individual pursuits, and sometimes they are used to team pursuits, but hardly ever are women accustomed to contact sports (except the occasional Easterners who play field hockey). And almost all martial arts styles require a great deal of physical contact. Men, who grow up playing football and basketball, are simply more likely to be used to physical contact. It can, however, be a great shock to women, and it can be very unnerving. Most of us are outraged at the thought of someone deliberately hitting us. We're simply not exposed to the possibility of it. Those of us who have had experiences with violence have tended to be or at least have been considered victims. If two men get in a barroom brawl, and one loses badly, his pride may be hurt, and his ribs cracked, but no one, least of all himself, really considers him a victim. Of course, on the scale of violence, this changes, but in a simple confrontation where punches are exchanged, the dynamics are much different for women than they are for men.

First, of course, there's the act of getting hit. This is hard to do without flinching or without feeling overwhelmed with fear or indecision or another emotion that makes reacting difficult. At lower belt levels, most martial arts styles restrict contact, so that it increases gradually as the practitioner becomes more comfortable with it. But even at the very beginning, the physical contact may be difficult, not because it is physically painful, but because mentally, emotionally, psychologically, we are not prepared for it. Getting hit also violates our sense of space. It makes us feel invaded and vulnerable. The martial arts often make it extremely clear that we are not nearly so brave and tough and strong as we had thought. But martial arts can make us even braver and tougher and stronger than before so that we become legitimately powerful. We become more powerful than we thought possible, if we give it a fair shot.

It is important in these first few experiences of contact to feel safe. It's okay to tell your partner, "I'm not comfortable with that level of contact," or to say, "Let's take this more slowly." Some people just learn to cope faster and some people aren't bothered at all by the physicality. Fear of contact, of course, is not simply a woman's problem. I once reduced a man to tears because as I was demonstrating a reverse kick, I touched his uniform with my foot (exhibiting, I thought, excellent technique and exquisite control). He gasped, "I'm just a yellow belt — no contact please!" And I immediately apologized and felt bad for having caused him distress. He was simply not used to having his space violated. So it is not that we are necessarily afraid of getting hurt—the main problem is we don't know what to expect. And we don't know what to do. I remember when I first started sparring, I got kicked in the hip (below the legal target area) and went to the women's locker room after class to shed some tears. One of the women, a black belt, took my distress seriously and made an effort to remind my partner to spar with better control.

What this means is to give yourself time to learn and permission to be distressed. It's part of the process. Then, when you are no longer affected by the contact, don't forget what it was like when you first started. This empathy is valuable for the other martial artists who come up through the ranks after you. Whether they are adults or children, female or male, they'll be happy to have your understanding.

Although I felt terrified when my partner kicked my hip when I was just a beginner, the fact that I was taken seriously helped me to develop the confidence that I wouldn't get hurt, that at this school, they didn't expect you to come equipped with the ability to brawl, and that your concerns would be taken seriously, so that you would actually be prevented from getting hurt. This wasn't of course exactly true, but it was reassuring for me.

Now I am a bit amused at how badly I responded to that kick. I've sparred men whose jump reverse kicks, even when blocked, move me back three feet and knock the wind out of me. Crazily enough, that just invigorates me more and makes me want the opportunity to blast may partner.

After a while, you realize that you can get hit, and you can even get hit pretty hard and it doesn't have to affect you. I've broken my hand and my arm, gotten contusions the size of dinner plates and still continued to spar. When I broke my arm, I sparred six more two minute matches, went home and graded papers and waited until the following afternoon to find out why my arm was bothering me. This wasn't bravado (well, maybe a little) so much as simply learning to let physical contact and the inevitable bumps and bruises happen, and not get too worked up over it. Although I had considerable pain, I also learned that having pain did not mean I immediately needed to stop what I was doing. This is not to say that you should continue working out if you have hurt yourself, which is not only stupid, but actually quite dangerous—I simply mean I realized that if I were actually in a fight and got hit or hurt, I wouldn't be so disoriented that I couldn't respond. I learned that it is stupid to spar with a broken arm but I also learned that you could.

When my arm was still in a cast, I continued a modified form of training. Why not spar when your arm is in a cast? Aren't people more likely to try to take advantage of you when you already appear to be more vulnerable than usual? I learned that even if I could only spar with one arm or one hand, I could be successful. There might be a time when I need that skill. More likely the confidence it gave me will be used in other ways. Perhaps some other task will seem overwhelming or impossible, until I remind myself that I am the one who can win a sparring match with one arm tied behind her back (well, not exactly).

Physical contact requires getting used to, so spend time doing it under controlled conditions. Have a friend grab your wrist while you practice a self-defense technique. Have your lover do a (gentle) chokehold while you decide what techniques can be used to your advantage. The more you work with people who are touching, grappling, grabbing or punching you, the more at ease you will become, and the sooner you will become so at ease. You'll also learn to respond much more quickly than usual because you'll be practicing often.

Another advantage to working with a wide variety of people is that you will become used to many different methods of attack and you'll learn many different methods of defense and counterattack. Often, we are taught techniques that would work well if we were men fighting other men. However, we are not. I remember working on one self-defense technique that worked like a charm against my partner, a woman my size. But when we rotated partners, and my new partner was a gangly 6 foot tall man with an attitude, the technique was absolutely worthless. I basically had to jump up and down on my tiptoes to do the technique. This is not an effective weapon, jumping up and down on your tiptoes, unless you wish to distract your opponent by amusing him so much he lets go and asks for additional jokes.

From this I learned my golden rule: women do not get attacked by other women who plan to mug them. At least, this is not the primary threat to women today. Women get attacked by men who wish to mug them or perhaps commit other crimes, such as rape. Men tend to be taller and heavier than women, so I should spend my time not training to fight someone my own size, but rather to fight someone a lot bigger than I am.

The other part of the golden rule is this: as infrequently as women attack and mug women, strange men attack and rape women at random. For women, the greatest threat is not some masked assailant in the bushes, but is in fact the men we know. The better we know them, the more dangerous they may be to us.

It is comforting to know when you are out on a date that if you say no to your date, you can back it up with a pretty powerful right cross, should you need to. A black belt friend whose 17-year-old daughter is also a black belt recently confided in me that as much as she worried about her daughter when she was out with friends or on a date, she always had the comfort of knowing her daughter was more prepared for anything that might happen than any of the other daughters of other people in the neighborhood.

This does not mean of course that we can be reckless and cavalier, certain of our ability to confront and destroy all attackers. It doesn't mean that a man won't succeed in hurting us if he tries. What it does mean, and this gives me comfort, is that he'll have more broken ribs after we're through than he had before. He'll wish he'd picked on someone else and hadn't tangled with me.

It's these thoughts that should help you become accustomed to contact. As you learn more, you may become, as I did, very angry that you were raised to be such a nice girl in a society that is this violent towards nice girls. If you find that this anger resides also in you, repeat the mantra: my parents wanted what was best for me. My parents didn't know any better.

I learned, as many women do, that much of our politeness stems not from courtesy but from fear. If we assert ourselves, we always wonder: if I have to go toe to toe with this person, will I survive? After some training, you realize that you don't assert yourself not because you're nice. You don't assert yourself because you are scared.

I remember six months after I began training, I told this huge guy at work to sit down and quit interrupting me when I spoke. And suddenly my palms were sweating (why on earth would I challenge this guy who could squash me just by sitting on me?) Then I realized that I had martial arts training. I was a bit arrogant. Everyone with six months' training is just a tad dangerous—to themselves. If he wanted to come after me, fine. After I punched him in the nose, I'd sidekick him in the groin. Then I'd sweep his leg and push him down and jump up and down on his gut. Then—but of course, no one threw a punch. The guy sat down and shut up. He never interrupted me again.

But while overcoming the mental blocks about taking hits, or in the case of some martial arts, hitting the floor or the mat, we have another difficulty to overcome. And that is hitting other people. Most women simply haven't gotten into fist fights. They may have been hit or slapped before, but they probably haven't punched back. This, for me, was even tougher than getting hit. I actually could not hit another person. Not another living creature with as much right not to get hit as me! My punches, in sparring, always landed about eighteen inches from the target. My kicks did too, but whether that was psychological or simply that I couldn't kick worth a darn at first, I don't know. As time went by, partners encouraged me to touch them with my punches. "Go ahead," they'd say, "Punch me!" Yeah, right. "I know you'll use good control," they'd say. But that wasn't really the problem. The problem wasn't that I was concerned about how hard I might hit them. The problem was hitting them at all. The problem was nice girls like me don't go around hitting people. Bottom line: ultimately I lacked confidence—maybe I would hurt someone, maybe I would make someone mad, maybe I would look foolish, maybe I would hurt myself, maybe I didn't have what it took to be a good martial artist, and if I really gave everything my best shot and found out I wasn't good enough—what then?

A few black belt women worked with me. They'd just stand there and make me punch them. Then we would spar a bit and then my partner would stop and make me punch her some more. This worked and I felt much better about myself. And just when I felt confident, I punched a partner too hard and hurt him. He kept walking into my reverse punch and I kept trying to pull it but to no avail. The following day my instructor took me aside and said I had cracked my partner's ribs. I was appalled. I stammered, I apologized, I explained how the match had gone, how the deed had been done, and then I couldn't bear to strike another person again. I really lost my nerve. I was just ready to test for my brown belt and I couldn't bring myself to spar confidently. I was nervous. I worked too slowly to hurt anyone. I didn't dare do any techniques to their fullest. I wouldn't try anything but the most basic techniques that I had complete faith in, that I could execute eighteen inches away from the other person. In short, I felt like a white belt again, only more miserable because I had actually hurt someone, I had no control, and on and on.

One of the female black belts said, "You know, people do get hurt by accident here. It's not ballet." And this I knew to be true, because I had already broken my hand by then, throwing a punch that was blocked. And she had a good point. Accidents happen. Even very good martial artists can hurt people without meaning to. Anyone who takes up martial arts training has to know it's not exactly low impact water aerobics. Still, I'd hurt someone and I couldn't spar. I didn't want to spar. I sparred only half-heartedly.

Then some of the guys got in the picture, telling me to go harder, that they could take it. This helped, but not much. After all, it was a guy's ribs I had broken, not a small woman's, not a kid's, a full-grown adult man who said I didn't have any control.

There was no quick solution to this problem but lots of practice. I practiced controlled punching and kicking on the heavy bag until I could do it with my eyes closed. This helped my training. And eventually I overcame my reluctance to spar. After a few months, it was again my favorite part of martial arts training. But I've never forgotten that you can hurt people, and that gives me a greater respect for the art and my ability to use it and control it. Many months later, a group of women were talking in the locker room after class. "Do you know what happened to Joe?" one was asking. She explained to me, "Joe was this real arrogant brown belt who was a real bully. He'd always go real hard against the women and if they'd complain he'd get all—you know, why are they here if they can't take it—but did he ever go hard against someone his own size and skill level? Oh, no. Only people smaller than him."

I shook my head. Too bad, I thought, that you could get to be a brown belt in a martial art and still not understand what it was about.

"Are you talking about Joe Smith?" another woman asked, "He's the idiot who took out my knee." Slowly, realization dawned on me.

"I know what happened to Joe Smith," I said, "I broke his ribs. He hasn't been back since."

Occasionally, justice is served in the martial arts, and though I was still wrong and at fault for not using better control and for causing an injury, I felt oddly relieved. It was somehow appropriate that I, who didn't know the man's background, actually served to help him understand what it was like when your partner sparred too hard, with too much skill against an opponent who was less skilled. This ability to punch, kick and otherwise invade the space of someone else is an important one. Not just for martial arts and not just to defend yourself against the stranger on the street who wants to hurt you. More women are injured and killed by their male relatives and loved ones than are hurt or killed by any other means. The greatest threat to a woman's survival is her father, brother, lover, husband, boyfriend, neighbor. In probably that order. When married women are murdered, the police always suspect the husband first, for he is usually the one who has done it. Most of us know the psychology of an abusive relationship is very complex. It is not so simple as a barroom brawl where winners and losers are decided in the exchange of a few punches and then everyone goes home to sleep it off.

But knowing how to punch another person, even a person you know and like, such as your sparring partner, is a wonderful skill. I've often wondered how many abusive relationships would never have gotten started if when he threw that first punch she'd blocked and countered hard to the solar plexus. Or the groin. Or how many date rapes could be avoided if when she said no, she had an elbow smash to the nose all ready to go. The martial arts emphasize three kinds of fighting situations: those where you simply block the attack and everyone walks away; those where you block the attack, but since the attacker isn't going to just walk away, you also control the attacker (think of his arm twisted behind his back; he isn't going to die of it, but he isn't going anywhere, either), and finally, the most physical confrontation when you not only block or escape an attack, but you also counter attack to make the opponent stop—to make the opponent unable to continue. (That arm you've got twisted behind his back? Go ahead and break it). The third is reserved for those rare situations that can usually be avoided if people simply use good sense. The first two are far more common. Someone grabs your shoulder, you twist free and continue walking. No one gets hurt, everyone leaves everyone else alone. Someone grabs your shoulder and you swing your arm around to immobilize his elbow, which, with a carefully placed strike, you could hurt very very badly. But you don't because everyone decides to leave each other alone.

Because women are likely to know their attacker, these first two abilities are essential. You may never want to see that boyfriend again, but you don't necessarily want to kill him. While he may deserve it, you don't really want to stand trial (do you?) Thus, the techniques that work against bigger and taller men and the techniques you can do to stop an attack without necessarily maiming the attacker for life are the techniques most useful in real life for real women.

But the martial arts aren't just about what physical confrontations might happen someday. There's a whole lot more to it, as you'll discover. Once you have become confident of your physical skills, you'll discover mental and emotional changes as well. You'll find yourself becoming a better person, braver and stronger in many ways. You just have to stick with it, even at those times when it seems overwhelming.

4

Self-Defense

Many women begin taking martial arts classes as a means of self-defense. They may also see it as a way to control weight and improve fitness, but a big reason, almost always, is that element of self-defense.

First, a disclaimer. As much as a martial art is about protecting yourself and your loved ones from harm, it's about many other things as well. It's about developing character, and living prudently, with integrity. It has a sport side. It has spiritual, mental and emotional aspects—at least for many people. One blue belt woman, when asked at a rank promotion test what had changed about her since she began martial arts training, said simply, "I've gotten taller." It wasn't exactly what she had intended to say, or how she wanted to answer the question, but we all understood anyway. All of us women who have earned black belts have, in the process, gotten taller too. If all you really want to know is rape prevention and self-defense, there are plenty of clinics and seminars that will teach you the basics of street fighting.

One of my head instructors, a woman, started training when she was 19. I started when I was 27. I've often said, ruefully, if only I'd started earlier in life, it wouldn't have been so hard to get and remain flexible. It was just a few months ago I learned that she'd never felt like it was an advantage to start young—she hadn't been flexible either and she was afraid, having focused almost exclusively on the sport aspect, that she might have missed something of value. In fact, extremely skilled athletes do report that they feel they're skipping or missing something because they focus so exclusively on the physical challenges of the sport. For those who must wait months for every quarter inch improvement in flexibility, seeing beyond the physical is much simpler. Learning the lessons has more meaning to someone who has to learn perseverance in order to break a board than for someone who can do it easily.

But one very important aspect of martial arts training *is* self-defense. Most martial arts programs split their training formally and informally into different areas. Techniques practice is repetitive practice of the techniques of the art, such as certain throws, sweeps, or kicks or punches that serve as the basis of the style.

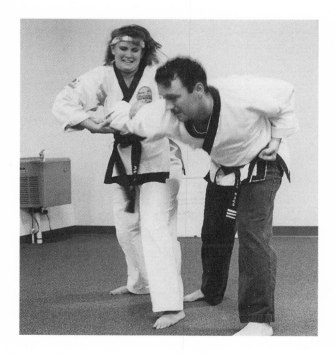

Self-defense is an integral part of all martial arts classes.

Body conditioning may also be worked in, usually through aerobic exercise and calisthenics. Forms, often called kata or hyung, may also demand attention. Learning and performing the forms correctly helps practitioners learn their techniques and gives them practice in stringing different techniques together. Sparring, a controlled fighting situation, is an opportunity for individuals to develop their own style of fighting and encourages the use of diverse strategies and tactics. It also helps students identify their strengths and weaknesses in a safe, carefully-controlled environment. In many cases, no contact to the head is allowed. No blows to the back, the legs, the groin and the hips are allowed. Often, hand techniques are limited, and frequently, throws aren't allowed. All these rules ensure a challenging yet fun experience without people getting hurt all the time.

The person sparring under controlled conditions, equipped with sparring gear, limited to certain techniques and target areas and restricted to a two-minute match is operating under an entirely different set of rules than exist in the outside world, where if someone wants to steal your purse, they're perfectly able to kick you in the knees. Then, too, of course, you can kick the attacker in the knees. But this is where self-defense training comes in. Almost every martial art has a set of self-defense techniques that apply to the kinds of circumstances one might find on the street. Thus, while flashy high jumping kicks might help you score points in a martial arts competition, they're strictly discouraged in self-defense situations.

However, most martial arts base their self-defense techniques on what works for men. To use these techniques successfully, women often need to modify them. What works on an attacker who is about your size and height may not work on one heavier and taller than you.

One person I used to train with must have weighed twice what I did. He was at least 260 or 270. He'd been a boxer, and he was a bit fat, but mostly he was tall, muscular, and because of his training, deceptively fast. A sidekick to his solar plexus didn't even make him grunt. *I'd* end up falling over, not him. Since he was good with his hands—jabs, crosses, hooks—I couldn't go inside and jam him, as I often do men (Their height is an advantage for them at kicking range, but a disadvantage at punching range). Sparring him was so difficult I often wondered what I'd do if I met someone like him on the street. After much trial and error, I learned that if I wanted to defend against someone like him, I was going to have to attack his knees. Even if I had wanted to attack his face (a punch or a palm strike to the nose or Adam's apple can really dispirit a person), I didn't want to try punching high because he was so good inside. For me to get that close to his punches would be stupid. But his knees—that was his vulnerable spot. But since his thighs were so massive, a direct kick to the knee might not work, especially if it turned out to be not completely on target. It would have to be perfectly placed with just the right amount of power to work. Too high and the blow would be absorbed by that massive thigh. Too low and I'd be jabbing at his calf, which he could just brush off. It wouldn't unbalance him.

But what about a sweeping kick to the back of his knee? Hard to block, hard to see coming. If it went too high, it could still force his knee to buckle, especially if it landed with enough force. A little too low would still take his leg out from under him. So my self-defense would be to roundhouse (sweep) kick hard to the back of the knee while pushing his body in the opposite direction. His knee would buckle forward and his body would fall backward, just like a hinge, and once he was on the ground, I could stomp on him or jump up and down on his torso if I wanted to, or, more prudently, walk quickly away in the opposite direction.

But although I had the leisure to study this problem at length (it took a little over four years to perfect), effective self-defense techniques can be acquired and used to good effort in a much shorter period of time.

Self-Defense and Your Life-style

For self-defense purposes, you should sit down and take some time to consider your life-style, personality and inclinations. This will be helpful in developing an arsenal of techniques that can be used in many self-defense scenarios.

Consider, first of all, how you spend the majority of your time. Are you a professional in a suit and heels? The skirt might give you some options (trust me, modesty is not a consideration during self-defense), since you might be able to perform different kicks with it on. But the heels will be a problem when it comes to kicking. I wouldn't want to try to pivot in four inch heels. However, they are a great asset for stomping, since the point of pressure is the heel, a relatively small area; stomp with a heel like that and you could puncture someone's foot. This is more helpful than stomping with only a tennis shoe to aid you.

My style, Tae Kwon Do, emphasizes kicks. But since I am self-employed and spend a lot of time out in the mud with my dogs, I wear jeans and sweatshirts. My feet are almost always bare except when I have to wear shoes and then I put on moccasins or loafers. Jeans restrict my ability to do kicks, but since I train in bare feet, all of that barefoot training will be of use when I have to defend myself out in the mud in my barefeet. Instead of trying to do sidekicks, which might be difficult given the tight fit of the jeans I prefer, I might instead rely on sweep type kicks, turning my body, not just my hip. Since my tops are always loose and roomy, I have plenty of opportunity and ability to use hand and elbow techniques. Also, if I have my loafers on, I can still do sweep kicks, and I'll probably be even less likely to injure my foot since the leather should protect it slightly.

It is not a bad idea to practice some of your best techniques while wearing the clothes you wear most frequently. This will help you to see what kind of self- defense techniques will be most viable.

Keep in mind that long heavy coats will get in the way of kicks. Material that drapes is easy to get hold of, and it may not be easy for you to simply pull away, letting the fabric tear. This you might be able to do in a cotton blouse, but not in a long suede coat. Some of today's synthetics are really tough. So you might have to contend with grips and grabs that are more difficult than usual to escape from.

Consider other aspects of your life style. Do you always have three bags of groceries, two kids and a dog in tow? Do any of them know what to do if you're approached or accosted by a stranger? Will they respond quickly to your commands? Will you be distracted by your concern for your loved ones? What can you do about this ahead of time?

If your children are old enough to learn about protecting themselves, have a serious conversation about what they should do when they're alone.

But also talk about what they should do if someone approaches them when they're with Mom. This changes their whole understanding of a threat and the appropriate response to it. They may see you as all-knowing and all-protecting, confident that you will take care of them. And while it is important that they can trust you this way, they also must know what to do to help you take care of them, as well as what to do if you can't take care of them. Do you know what you would do if you had to protect them and yourself at the same time? Don't scare the poor kids to death—or yourself either—but do think about it. As for the dog, I've always said a good big dog is worth any number of armed men at my side, but unless you are going to train it professionally as a guard dog, and then, therefore, *not* as a companion or family pet, do not depend on your dog to do anything but lick a deranged criminal. It is imperative that your dog can sit and stay with or without your hand on its collar or leash. If it wants to take a chunk out of the attacker's left thigh, let the dog go for it. But more likely than not, the dog will only serve to get in your way and distract you. A dog is a good deterrent only. If you can command your dog to sit and stay, and it does, your potential assailant may begin to wonder what else you have trained it to do. Also, a dog that is sitting and staying during a potential confrontation is simply one less distraction you need to worry about.

Myself, I have an adorable Alaskan malamute cross. She looks like a timber wolf, which is just exactly what you want your dog to look like if you have one for the reason of protecting you. My dog is also lean and wiry like a wolf since she doesn't each much and she has so much energy she's bouncing off the walls all the time. She has two drawbacks. One, she's never met a stranger. All people and all animals are long-lost friends to her. Second, she has no more common sense than a snail. I could be screaming for mercy and she'd be out in the yard chasing her tail, looking up only infrequently to see if the rabbit, which she has failed to catch for two years, is around anywhere.

However, since she wants to meet and lick everyone, she must be restrained. When I restrain her and she nonetheless pulls forward, it looks exactly as if she is getting ready to rip someone's throat out. This has intimidated no end of pizza delivery guys. At any rate, I encourage her behavior when salespeople come to the door. Although she is not supposed to jump up, she does jump up on the front window when someone rings the doorbell. A visitor only sees a very tall wolf (she is, of course, standing on a table to look out the window.) Plenty of salespeople haven't even bothered to wait for me to come answer the door. One time, she escaped my clutches and jumped on the Fed Ex guy, who went still as a statue and turned completely pale. I pulled her off after she'd slurped a lick or two across the Fed Ex guy's face. He said, "Good thing she's friendly," and I said sternly, "You're lucky. She's usually not."

Since I am alone most of the time, I prefer the world to think that I life with a savage wolf dog, so that a person with any sense would avoid my house. I recently adopted a Rottweiler pup who'd been abandoned. I'm fairly sure people will confuse her with a Doberman, and then even the insurance salespeople will refuse to ring the bell. But that does not mean my dogs make me safer. They're a deterrent, that's all. They'd be easy to shoot or poison should someone want to come into my house. But it is true that if given a choice, someone who intends to rob or harm you will look for a woman in a house without dogs, as opposed to a woman in a house with two big dogs.

But just because your kids and dogs can be distracting, this doesn't mean you should change your whole life-style and never take your kids and your dog to the same place at the same time. It only means that you should be aware of your habits and what you might have to do because of them. The one and only rule about confrontations and self-defense is that only the things that are alive are worth hanging onto and protecting. You must be perfectly willing to let your car go, your wedding ring go, your purse go, the antique brooch your late grandmother gave to you; you must be ready to let your groceries fall to the ground and that table lamp you have been saving up for over the past six months—you should be ready to smash it over a would-be assailant's head. The lovely leather coat your dear boyfriend gave you for Christmas—you'd better be prepared to rip it. These things have no value. It is important to keep that in mind.

Many women report that their reaction to an assault was delayed because they had shopping bags in their hands. Drop them! Since women do most of the shopping and then all of the hauling and carrying indoors, we're sort of trained to get run over by kids and dogs and husbands while still retaining a tight grip on dinner. So experiment a bit. I once returned from the grocery store, got out of my car and on impulse dropped the grocery bags on the driveway and assumed a fighting stance. What the neighbors thought, I do not know. I did not ask. This would have worked

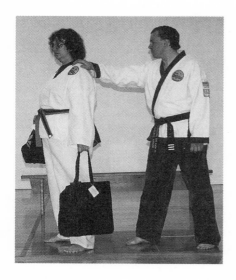

*Practicing realistic
scenarios, such
as the ones shown
here, can prepare
you to defend yourself
in a real life
confrontation.*

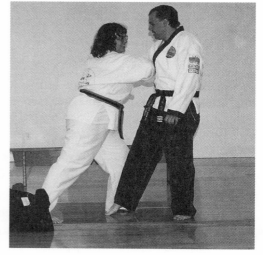

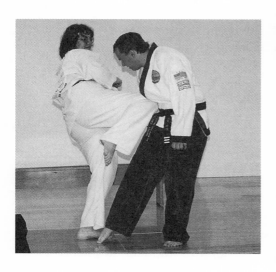

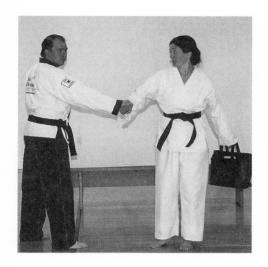

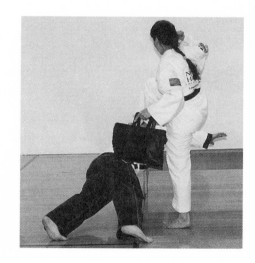

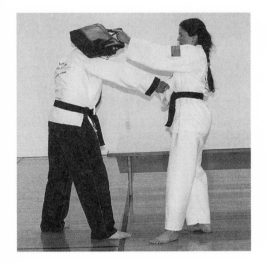

better if I had also dropped my purse, but it was very satisfying. I cracked open the carton of milk and squashed some rolls, but that's all. And I showed myself that I could be ready to defend myself at almost any time.

As you assess your life-style, don't leave out things like terrain. My yard is all level and grassy, so I wouldn't be afraid fighting out there. My house is carpeted just like my training hall, so I'm comfortable there, too. But as I discover every winter, even grass is slippery in the snow and ice. So I always practice falling in the winter so I won't be afraid of it. You probably don't want to go to the ground with an assailant unless you are a skilled grappler, and then only if it's one-on-one. But learning to fall is always a good idea—then if you do fall, you won't be completely unnerved and disoriented.

In self-defense, learning how to take a punch is essential. Often, women don't put up much of a fight because the first blow disorients them so much. So always be ready to take a hard knock and then respond.

Considering Scenarios

In addition to considering terrain—not just around your house but where you work, as well—consider your other habits. Do you drive a lot? Do you know what to do if someone bumps you from behind? Do you visit a lot of different places in the course of a day? Does your office building become a ghost town after five? Do you know where the closest safe place is—gas station, police station? Do you know what to do if your car won't start? If you blow out a tire, can you change it? Why not? Do you know when it's safe to drive a damaged car and when this may be extremely dangerous? For instance, if you have a flat tire, you can drive on the rim until you reach a lighted area with people and a phone. You may have to replace the wheel (but remember, the only things worth worrying about are the things that are alive). But if your oil pressure suddenly plummets because of a torn hose or an insecurely fastened plug? Your engine could seize up in moments, meaning that not only would you have a useless car and still not be in a safer environment, but you might also lose control of the vehicle and involve yourself in an accident. The best thing might be to lock all your doors, use your cell phone if you have one, and wait until you are more immediately threatened to try to move the vehicle.

You see, even your car is a terrain of sorts. What if you are at a stop light and someone attempts a car jacking? What martial arts techniques will you manage while seatbelted into place? Again, this isn't meant to suggest that not wearing a seat belt gives you greater freedom of movement so you shouldn't wear one, or that you should quit stopping at red lights. Just think about it for a few minutes and decide what you would do. Then get what you need (training, etc.) to be able to do it. You may never need this course of action, or when you do need it, this course of action might fail. But at least you won't have to live your life saying, I never thought it would happen to me and I didn't have the slightest idea what to do.

If you have martial arts skills, and think you'd use them for self-defense, also consider how much flexibility and power you might have on any given day. After I've warmed up and stretched a bit I can kick a 6'6" guy in the head, but I'd be lucky to hit chest high if I'm kicking cold. I can probably count on some adrenaline should someone choose to attack me, but probably not enough to kick 6'6" high. That's why I think of knees when I think of self-defense techniques. I also think of using hand techniques to an attacker's nose or eyes. Visualize this sort of thing. Can you really gouge someone's eyes, do you think? You might be better off aiming for the nose. Probably all of us can feel comfortable punching someone in the nose, whereas sticking your keys in an attacker's eyes, as some women's magazines suggest, seems a lot more difficult to do. And remember, you may know your attacker. I wouldn't mind punching my brother in the nose if he decided to slap me, but I seriously doubt I'd be able to take out his eyes. Plus, think of what the family would say.

Always be ready to do more than one technique. If you're going to fight, and I hope you are, you are going to have to fight like you mean it. If someone grabs your sleeve and you pull away, but he's stronger than you and he's still got hold of your sleeve, keep at it. Kick, bite, stomp. You must be persistent, you must use full force and you must commit yourself to the fight. In other words, you're going to have to mean it.

I used to work on this ax kick that I swear would knock the living daylights out of anyone unfortunate enough to get in the way of it. Unfortunately for me, I got it right about once in every five or six tries.

Otherwise, I'd end up bouncing my calf off the top of someone's shoulder. This would only irritate my partner, not impress him or her. One of my sparring partners once said, "OK, I'm an attacker, you've bounced your leg off my shoulder, which hurts, and now I'm mad." The thrust of this was, don't anger an attacker by slapping at him. Hurt him. Make him stop. Finish it, as we say. If it requires six techniques, fine, but do each technique as if this were the knockout punch. When I work on a technique that's complicated but otherwise powerful and a lot of fun, I ask myself, am I consistently doing this technique well enough to take someone out, or will I just anger someone? Techniques that I have not perfected I do not consider for personal self-defense (although I continue to practice them). As I grow proficient in a technique, I'll add it to my arsenal. A few years ago, I'd never have thought of using a jump reverse kick in a confrontation. Now I would. I'm confident enough that I'll land it right (or right enough) every time. I've gotten to the same point with a 360 degree kick I've been working on. But the spinning wheel kick I've known how to do since my second month of Tae Kwon Do lessons? Not a chance.

Weapons

Some people may not wish to rely only on their empty hand techniques for self-defense. Many people keep guns and knives. While these weapons can certainly dissuade a person from attacking you, they have limits as well. In households with children, there's always the danger of accidental shootings (in all households there's always the danger of accidental shootings, but these occur with frightening regularity in houses with children). There's also the danger of intentional shooting. Plain old-fashioned arguments with friends and relatives turn deadly when weapons are easily available. In the United States, a handgun is more likely to be used against a friend or family member than against a criminal or intruder. More ordinary people are shot with their own handguns than ever shoot dangerous attackers. Some people put the ammunition in one place and the gun itself in another to prevent children or others from accidentally firing the gun. But the likelihood of you being able to get the ammunition into the gun in time to stop an attacker is minimal. From the time you perceive a threat to the time it takes to get the gun from the dresser, the bullets from the closet, feed the bullets into the chamber, or the clip to the gun, as your hands are shaking—say, hasn't that crazy guy already knocked down your bedroom door? Wouldn't you have been better off calling 911 and hiding in the closet?

On occasion, I've been at gatherings where people find out that I practice the martial arts and someone always says dismissively, "My Smith and Wesson'll beat your sidekick every time." I'm sure every martial artist has heard this comment at least once. I once put a chokehold on an idiot who said this and then asked him where his gun was so he could take me out. He complained that my "attack" was unfair. Unfair? Does he really believe a mugger is going to be fair? No, a criminal isn't likely to strike while you are in the middle of a cocktail party, but he will try to strike when you are at your most vulnerable, most unsuspecting and therefore at the greatest disadvantage. So unless you carry that gun strapped to your thigh all the time, it is fundamentally worthless to you. You might as well not have it at all since chances are it'll be used against you or someone you love long before it stops a rapist from climbing in through your bedroom window.

Knives and other such weapons have the same drawbacks. They're worse to use than guns since they are much more personal. I once attended a knife training seminar in which I learned all the grisly ways to use a knife against an attacker, the primary technique being to shove the knife into the attacker's armpit, and, using a pumping action, sever the artery there. I came away from that seminar knowing that I could never use a knife against someone. So don't feel confident that you have the cleaver under your mattress unless you are convinced that you'd use it, and have been trained in how to use it. Just jabbing at someone with a knife is not going to impress him (or her). More likely you'll just make the person angry. Also, you don't want someone to use your knife on you. You'd rather have them use your handgun on you. Trust me. In the case of weapons like these, you must be certain they are readily available without being so available your kid or your mom will get hurt with it, and you must commit yourself to training with the weapon until you have mastered using it. Once you have done so, you will still need to continue taking lessons or practicing the use of the weapon, because like all else, it is much too easy to forget how.

But what if your attacker has a weapon, which, considering the state of the world, is not entirely unrealistic? Empty handed training against weapons is reserved usually for the highest level of students at most martial arts schools. It is dangerous to do, and it is also dangerous to teach students what to do against a gun and then have them go forth falsely thinking that they can disarm any mugger with a .38. Probably the best thing to do when you see a weapon is to run as fast as you can in the opposite direction. Handguns aren't very accurate against moving targets, especially beyond 100 feet. Knives, of course, are in-close weapons, and while they can be thrown they are even less accurate than guns and also much less deadly. No reason you can't continue running even if you've got a switchblade sticking out of the back of your upper arm. Beyond that, remember only the live things are worth hanging onto. This, too, is a time when you decide that the African violet and the goldfish, while certainly alive and deserving of continued life, won't miss it as much as you will.

A point about weapons. If a guy with a gun says he won't hurt you if you just do as he says, don't believe it. Please. You've never listened to a guy's lines before, have you? My personal philosophy is this: someone who has gone to the trouble to arm himself, and then has bothered to pick me out of the crowd and grab me—this is a person who is intent on having his way, whatever that might be. He can have my purse or my car, but he doesn't get to have me along with it. A long time ago I decided that armed men would kill you or would not kill you pretty much regardless of what you did. So my decision was, would I rather be murdered trying to run away, or would I rather be raped and tortured for sixteen days and then murdered? You can see how much simpler the decision is when you are realistic.

Again, however, remember that women are attacked by men they know, and women are murdered by men they know much more frequently than they are injured or murdered by strangers. If it is clear to all the men in your life always that you will kick the living tar out of them should they try to hurt you, you are one very large step ahead of your sisters who are still looking for polite ways to say, "please stop hurting me."

Being Prepared

Self-defense, then, is a matter of taking care in your relationships too. And taking care of yourself. Stay fit and alert, refrain from drinking to drunkenness and the like, and you'll find yourself in far fewer dangerous situations.

As you consider your self-defense needs, remember that the situations you may encounter will vary tremendously. It's one thing if a person just hassles you a bit. Maybe another driver on the road tries to intimidate you a little. While that can be a little scary, it is quite different from being followed or physically or verbally threatened. Women seem more worried about offending strangers than they are about putting themselves in dangerous situations. If you're on an elevator and a creepy guy gets in with you, why on earth risk it when your impulse is to get out and wait for the next elevator? So the creepy-looking guy gets insulted. Would you rather have your purse stolen or get assaulted? Nine people out of ten understand just how you feel and the tenth will think you forgot your briefcase. You can even make a remark if you'd feel more comfortable— "Better check to see if I turned off my headlights." The same goes for modesty. A convicted serial rapist once said he'd found it amazingly simple to assault women if the first thing he did was simply push their skirt up or pull their blouse open. They were so preoccupied trying to remain modestly covered that they didn't fight back the way they might have. Wouldn't you rather be slightly embarrassed by running out in public in a torn skirt than to have to live with having been raped—or perhaps not even having that option? There is nothing wrong with insulting people, nothing wrong with being seen in your underwear and certainly nothing wrong with screaming, fighting, biting and gouging your way out of a dangerous situation if the alternative is to be hurt.

You should take the time to cultivate your powers of observation. This can actually be a fun exercise. Be aware of your surroundings. Ask yourself, Where are the exits? Where are the elevators and stairwells? Where do the halls or roads lead? Take the time to learn about the areas you are in most often. Always exercise extreme caution when you are in a situation that is unfamiliar to you. My husband is also a black belt in Tae Kwon Do, and yet he is almost completely oblivious to his surroundings. There are no bad parts of town to him, just some poor folks who live in one area and some richer folks who live in another, and folks is folks. While I admire his attitude in many ways, it scares me to death. Partly I think this is related to gender. All he can imagine is that someone might steal his wallet or his car and he can manage okay if that happens. But women are told repeatedly that the mugger won't stop there. They're repeatedly told that they'll be dragged off to an abandoned warehouse, repeatedly raped and then left to die an agonizingly slow death. Not quite as harmless a picture as getting your wallet stolen, is it?

My husband used to make light of my discomfort until I spelled it out to him and mentioned that only an insensitive clod would ridicule those fears. More than that, though, I do consider it a town/country difference. He was raised in the country by parents who never locked their doors and nothing bad ever happened to them. They left car keys in the ignition, and the cars weren't stolen. Growing up in the city, where everything that wasn't fitted with an alarm and nailed down was fair game, I had a slightly different upbringing. People, even neighbors, did not know each other and certainly did not look out for each other. Before I was allowed to go out at night, I was expected to repeat the mantra: the car will remain full of gasoline so that I'll always have plenty to get somewhere. The car doors will remain locked at all times except for the moment I am actually entering or exiting the vehicle. I'll check for people hiding in the backseat before I get into the car. Sometimes I thought it was too much, but nothing too bad ever happened to me, though I had a couple scares. So I think my husband and his country folk are just plain foolish because what's at stake is not only the silver locked up in the dining room.

Some people carry pepper spray or mace or whatever their state says is legal to carry. (You can carry a concealed weapon in more states than you can carry mace.) Like guns and knives, it is foolish to rely on your pepper spray to be there all the time. It also takes practice to use, though you might not think so. You'll have to get your purse opened and remove the can, find the nozzle and the button—what if the attacker grabbed your purse first thing and tossed it aside? And when you spray that stuff, what if in your nervousness you turned the nozzle toward yourself? Or you sprayed into a stiff wind? It is simply more sensible to be prepared to use the one thing you'll always have, which is yourself. These other weapons may make good supplemental choices, but they should not be your primary defense. More importantly, they should never be your only defense.

Many women think that having a male companion, a live-in lover, or a husband, will keep them safe. It's an old stereotype that whenever the wife hears a scary noise downstairs she sends the husband to investigate. Our house could be felled by an earthquake and my husband would sleep through it, so I don't count on him protecting me from harm.

The point has been driven home to me so many times that I've decided that women aren't afraid of being lonely, which is commonly cited as the reason they don't leave bad relationships. Women are afraid of being alone, and not just emotionally but physically, because they are unprepared to take care of themselves on any count. Now that's more foolish than my in-laws leaving the keys to the car in the ignition. Men aren't all that valuable of a deterrent. Get a dog. First of all, what happens when the man you live with is the one who threatens you? Now what? What about the times when he is not there to "protect" you—say during the times when you're at work?

You can't stay attached to his hip and have a healthy relationship. Those times when he can't be there—he's at work, on a business trip, you get home earlier than he does, you're out alone doing some Christmas shopping? What about those times? Nothing is going to happen to you then? And just what is it about the man in your life that makes him such a good guard? I have a rottweiler who sits for hours right next to me, ready to attack should anyone try to hurt me. (No, I never trained her to be a guard dog, she just turned out that way; as I said, trained guard dogs require constant attention and are more than the ordinary citizen can handle. They are not house pets or companions, and if the owner loses control over the dog, it can be dangerous to everyone nearby.) At any rate, my dog came by her guarding instinctively. She is simply happiest when sitting next to me and watching for attackers. The only drawback is that she is three months old and weighs about sixteen pounds. The lovely thing has the heart of a lion and she does think she's an even match for any attacker, but the fact is a sixteen pound puppy isn't much use for personal protection, and the fact is, most men aren't either. How many men have had to defend themselves and others?

How many actually know more than you do about how to throw a good punch? This was driven home to me once after I have been training in the martial arts for about eight months. I'd supplemented the conditioning workouts with weight training and swimming. So I was actually in better shape than I have ever been. I rented a canoe with a new boyfriend and ten minutes later he complained that he couldn't move the paddles another stroke, he was so sore. He was envious of the shape I was in. I really thought he was joking at first, because I was just beginning to enjoy it. But no, he meant it. So I'm supposed to find some guy who can't paddle half as much as I can, and I am supposed to be comforted in his presence and by his presence since he will protect me from all harm? Hah. The only person who I can count upon to save me is me.

Another incident helped assure me of this. I lived alone in one side of a duplex. One day I came home to find a photograph nailed to my front door. It was a picture of me, taken at a football game where there'd been 60,000 screaming fans. My face had been circled in black ink, heavily, and arrows were drawn on the picture pointing to me. There was no note (saw you at the game), no phone message (dropped off that photo, couldn't believe I spotted you in that crowd!), or anything of that nature. So I did what any sane woman who watches T.V. would do. I called my best friend and said I was being stalked. She empathized. Then I called the police and showed the idiot who arrived the photo, explained the situation, and was asked the question, "So this makes you nervous?" That is how hopelessly clueless male police officers are about crimes against women (I realize what I have described is not a crime, but it never even occurred to him that it could be a slightly scary thing to find nailed to your front door). I couldn't believe the question. No, I call the police every time people photograph me, just to share.

After I made it clear that the incident was disturbing, he said, "Report any suspicious activity and let us know if you start getting phone hang-ups, things like that." Then he said, "I wouldn't worry if I was you." In addition to the poor grammar, I was outraged at his attitude. Easy for him to say. They weren't going to find his body washed up on the bank of the river. His bad judgment wasn't going to make a bit of difference in his life, except he might get called upon to investigate a homicide—mine.

I also called a male friend, who also emphathized with me and further wanted to punch whoever had scared me. The only actual productive thing that happened is I got mad, told everyone to go away and started interviewing the neighbors. Had they seen anyone at my house? People always love to be involved in minor dramas this way. From them, I tracked down a car, a description of the person driving the car, and after further discussion with other people, including the friends of friends, I learned that it was a recent ex-lover who'd left the photo on my door. And while I might have suspected as much, it was helpful to have confirmed it. I reminded all the people who knew my former lover how poorly the police looked down on guys with long hair nailing photos to doors, and so the idiot never followed up on whatever it had been his intention to do. Even his roommate made fun of him, asking, "You been out leaving photos on doors again?" Nothing like a bit of public ridicule to discourage mean-spirited, vicious-minded men.

Through this informal network, I was able to learn the identity of the person who left an anonymous threat, remind him that even if it was just a prank, it could backfire and land him in court, and I managed to end any sort of nonsense before it really had a chance to get started. Who knows what would have happened otherwise? Probably absolutely nothing. But I would have spent a lot of time worrying and wondering, wringing my hands and feeling powerless and passive. I have a right not to be bothered and harassed in my own home, but I was the only one who was motivated enough to do anything about it. After feeling like a victim, an unwitting target, I went on the offensive and regained control. Just the investigation itself proved that I could do something about an attack even if it was subtle, indirect and anonymous.

Since you're going to rely primarily on yourself, you need to be able to handle the variety of situations that might arise. In addition to things like what would you do if you knew your attacker (perhaps it's your husband, or, as in my case, an ex-lover), you need to consider what you would do if an attacker were armed. You might even do some training for defense against weapons. In addition to your martial arts training, there are numerous rape prevention clinics and seminars that will help you learn to deal with an armed assailant. You should also be able to fight on the ground, although this is something you want to avoid at all costs, since fights that go to the ground are difficult to survive, let alone win. You need to think about which of your techniques can work when you're on the ground. Practice in different positions—on your back, then your stomach. Again, think of things like environment—climate, terrain, what you'll be wearing, where such a confrontation might take place.

Finally, you'll need to consider how you'd handle a scenario with multiple attackers. Grappling definitely won't work. Your goal is to survive, preferably intact, rather than to win, so escaping and running away should always be your goals.

For people who practice martial arts styles that use weapons, such as karate or escrima, the techniques you learn on the stick or nunchuks can actually be adapted to other weapons. Empty hand styles also have many techniques that are suitable to use with weapons. Think about the weapons that exist in your environment. Your hands and your feet are the obvious ones, as are things like the kitchen knives you may have. A heavy ceramic vase might work, as could an iron that might be swung and then thrown. In your office, you might have pens and pencils to gouge eyes or other sensitive areas, a phone to hit with, a letter opener, a heavy paperweight. Consider all the objects around you and their potential use. Even simple things, like the diamond engagement ring you don't wear to martial arts class because you're afraid it will scratch someone could be used. Scratching it across someone's face would hurt a bit, wouldn't it? What have you got in your car? A cell phone? A briefcase? Think of how you might use any or all of these things.

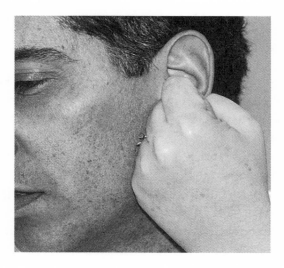

Even something as simple as a ring can become a painful weapon when used to strike to the sensitive areas of the face.

There are different categories of weapons, and weapons in each category have different purposes. There are those weapons that are used to distract—a fistful of sand, the scratching diamond ring, a box of files thrown toward someone. Then there are projectile weapons, such as the iron you swing on a cord and then throw. If you are a softball player and there's a softball handy, launch that. There are long range weapons—a broom handle to poke someone away from you, a garden rake, the like. Short range weapons include those that are about as long as an arm. Fireplace tools, for instance, work well as short range weapons—the poker makes a good choice. The ubiquitous baseball bat and golf club—these are certainly cliched, but it does hurt to get walloped on the head with a bat. There are bladed weapons, like knives, letter openers and the like. The garage is a handy place to find these kinds of weapons. Just remember if you use an environmental weapon, you must be certain your attacker won't be able to get it away from you, and you must be committed to using it. If you can't quite imagine gouging someone's eye out, then put the pens and pencils away and get out the baseball bat. Also remember that as you look around, spotting the potential weapons in your environment, that a potential attacker could do exactly the same thing. So even if you think the attacker does not have a weapon, it takes just a moment for him to acquire one.

Finally, remember your main goal: escape. All else is secondary to that. Escape, control and counter are the three degrees of self-defense, and the three levels of conflict. Each is more dangerous than the last, but doing nothing and being unprepared are perhaps the most dangerous acts of all.

Self-Defense Techniques

Once you've identified the possibilities in your life-style, it's time to move on to specific self-defense techniques for common situations. The most valuable techniques are those that can be used or modified to fit any of the three levels of conflict. For instance, if someone grabs your shoulder, and you pull away to free yourself, you are operating on the escape level. All you wish to do is escape from the attacker. You don't necessarily need to go beyond this. But let's say the attacker grabs your sleeve, you pull away and he grabs your sleeve again. That persistence has moved the conflict to another level. This time, when you pull your arm away, you'll trap his hand to control him. Again, you've moved to the control level of self-defense, but you still haven't injured anyone and you have kept the conflict within reasonable bounds.

But perhaps your attacker isn't ready to give up that easily. While you have his hand trapped, he kicks you. Now the attacker's persistence has moved the conflict to the next level, where you will have to counter with an attacking technique of your own to make the attacker back down. This third level is the most dangerous because it is where your conflict will turn into an out-and-out brawl. But you must be ready and willing to go to this level should it be necessary.

Of course, no encounter is going to be predictable. And it might be unwise in certain situations to simply try to escape without first stopping your attacker. But the point is that using deadly force on a man who simply grabbed your arm will get you into a great deal of trouble, even if you thought you were only defending yourself. Therefore, depending on the attacker's actions and persistence, you will need to be able to respond at different levels. Again, escape, control and counter are the levels of self-defense you need to be skilled at, so the best techniques are those that can be modified to suit each level.

Remember, too, as you learn self-defense techniques in your martial arts class, that not all techniques work well for women. Practice all of your self-defense techniques on men who are bigger and heavier than you, as well as on women who are more your size. It takes practice to adjust to different kinds of people.

The following self-defense techniques are examples of skills work for women against men, and can be modified for any of the three levels of conflict that have been discussed. Some attacks, such as the wrist grab, have a variety of defenses demonstrated, beginning with the simplest to learn, followed by more advanced variations. These scenarios should be considered examples only - real life confrontations are unpredictable and will not necessarily proceed as those demonstrated in the sample scenarios.

Self-Defense Against a Wrist Grab

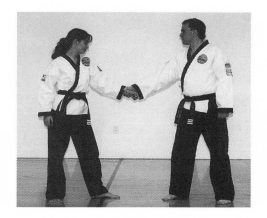

When an atacker grabs your left wrist with his right hand . . .

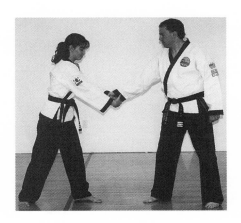

grasp your left hand tightly with your right hand . . .

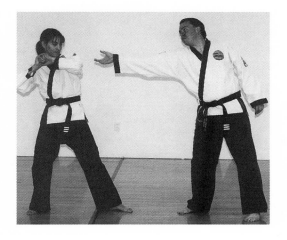

and quickly pull up and towards yourself.

Self-Defense Against a Wrist Grab

When the attacker grabs your left wrist with his right hand, lean backwards . . .

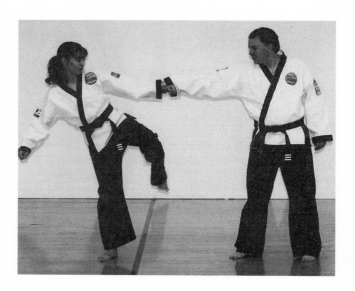

and deliver a left side kick to his ribs.

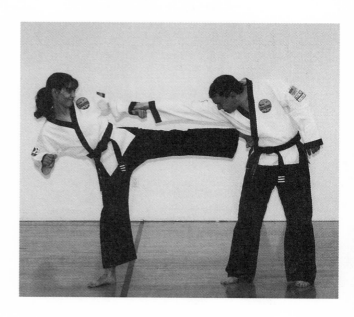

Self-Defense Against a Wrist Grab

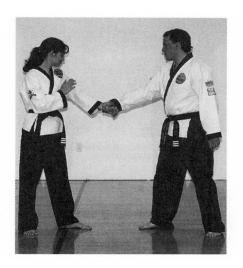

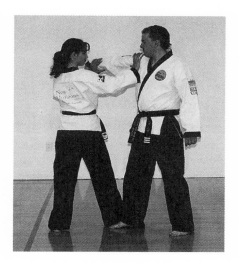

When the attacker grabs your left wrist with his right hand . . .

step toward him and place your right hand on his shoulder . . .

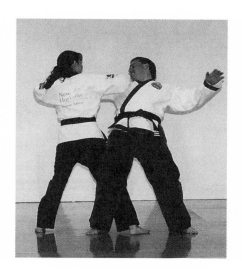

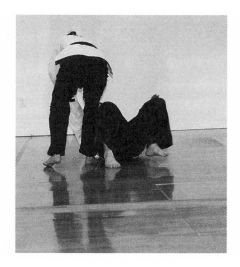

push him backward using your right leg to trip him.

When he falls to the ground, run away.

Self-Defense Against a Wrist Grab

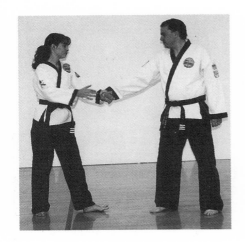

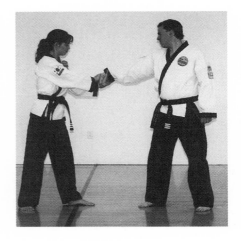

*If you cannot pull
free from a wrist grab . . .*

*turn your hand palm up. Cover the
attacker's hand with your hand.*

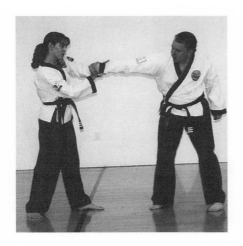

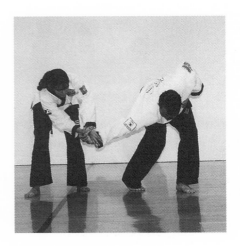

*Twist the attacker's
wrist clockwise . . .*

forcing him to the ground.

Self-Defense Against a Wrist Grab

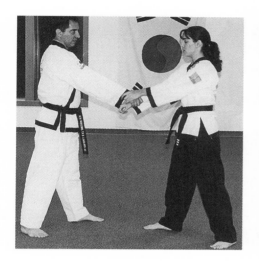

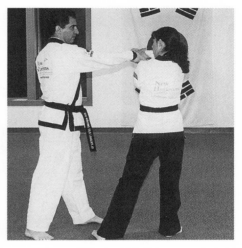

When the attacker grabs your right wrist grip it with your left hand.

Turn to your right while stepping away from the attacker.

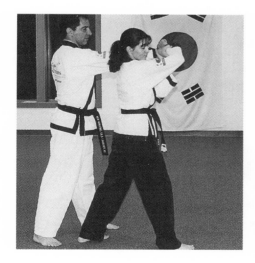

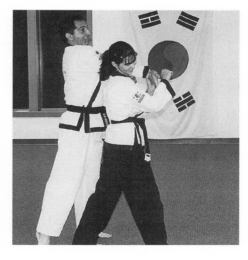

Pull his arm over your shoulder with his palm facing upward.

When his elbow is on your shoulder, pull his hand downward.

Self-Defense Against a Wrist Grab with Both Hands

When your right wrist is grabbed by two hands . . .

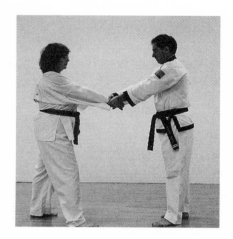

clasp your left and right hands together and pull up and over your shoulder.

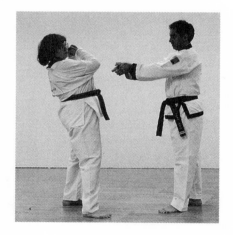

You can follow up with a backfist strike to the temple.

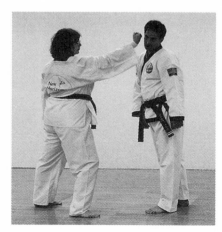

Self-Defense Against a Two-Wrist Grab

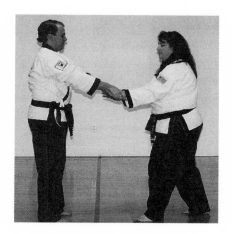

When both wrists are grabbed. . .

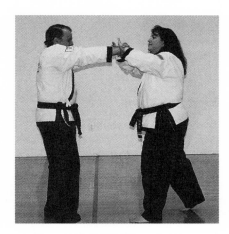

Swing your arms upward and twist your hand so you can grab his wrists.

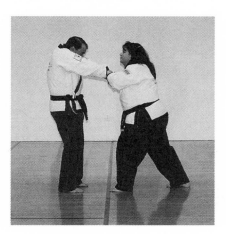

Step and push the attacker away.

Self-Defense Against a Two-Wrist Grab from Behind

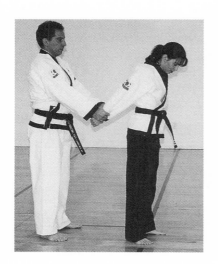

When both wrists are grasped from behind . . .

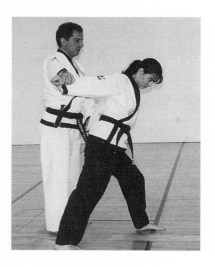

step backward and raise your arms while lowering your body.

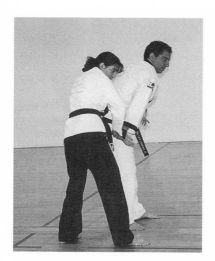

Jerk your arms down while moving away from the attacker.

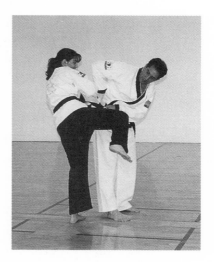

Follow with a knee strike to the stomach.

Self-Defense Against an Attack from Behind

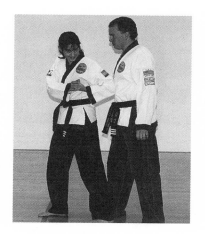

When threatened from behind, use an elbow strike to the solar plexus . . .

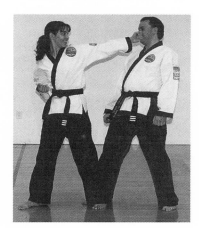

followed by a backfist to the face . . .

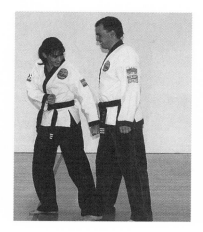

and a hammer fist to the groin.

Self-Defense Against a Sleeve Grab

When grabbed by the upper arm or sleeve . . .

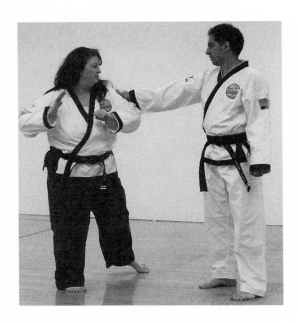

strike the attacker's face with your open palm.

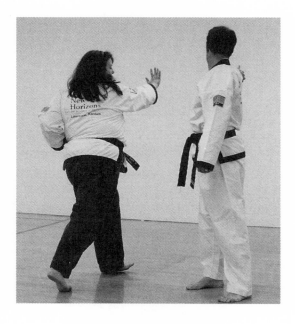

Self-Defense Against a Sleeve Grab

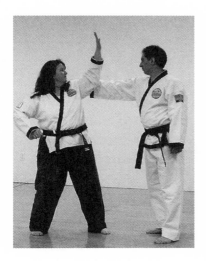

When grabbed by the sleeve, raise your arm.

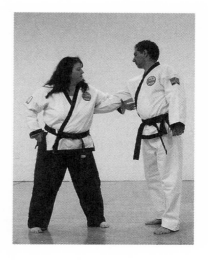

Wrap it around the attacker's arm just above the elbow.

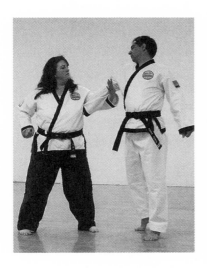

Lift the attacker to gain control.

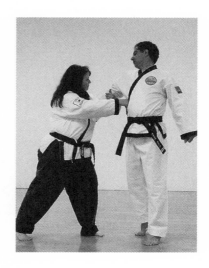

Strike to his exposed ribs.

Self-Defense Against a Sleeve Grab from Behind, Using a Weapon

When grabbed from behind while holding your keys . . .

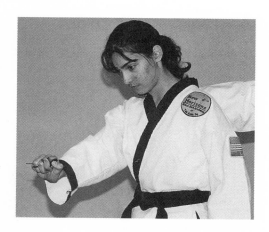

turn toward your attacker, lifting your arm above his arms . . .

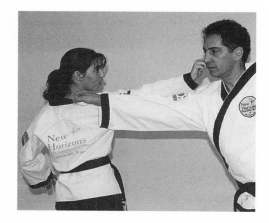

and strike to his face with your keys.

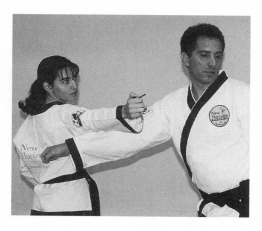

Self-Defense Against a Shirt/Lapel Grab

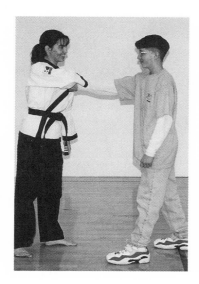

*When grabbed from
the front. . .*

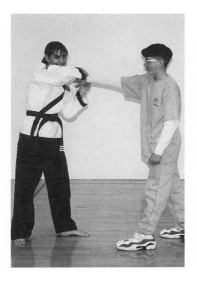

*grasp the attacker's hand
with both hands.*

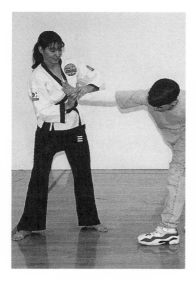

*Twist his hand over so his palm and
elbow are facing upward . . .*

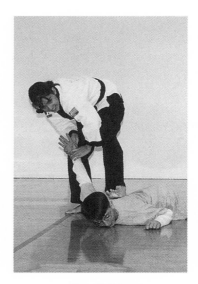

*and pull him
to the ground.*

Self-Defense Against a One-Arm Chokehold

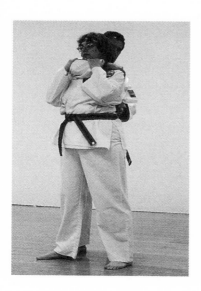

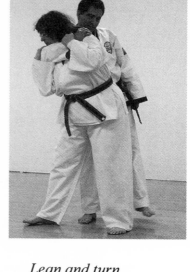

When choked from behind, grab the arm with both hands.

Lean and turn into the choke.

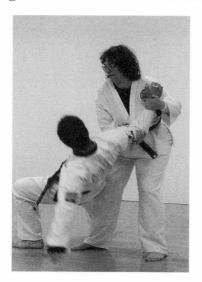

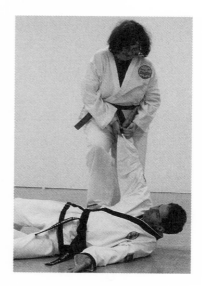

Keep turning and pull down on his arm to disrupt his blance.

Follow with a stomp kick to the ribs.

Self-Defense Against a Two-Handed Chokehold

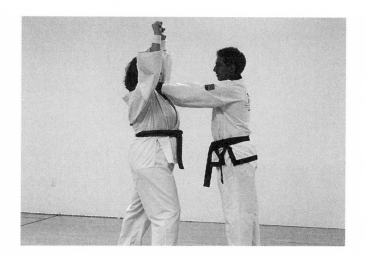

When choked from the front, lift both arms up over your head . . .

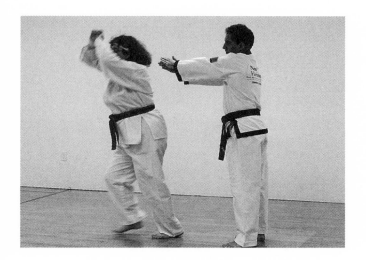

turn quickly and run away.

Self-Defense Against a Two-Handed Chokehold

When choked from the front . . .

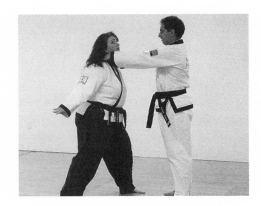

strike both of your attacker's sides with your open hands.

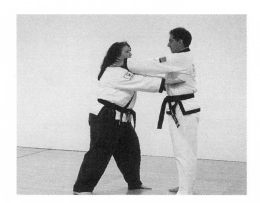

Raise your arms up between his arms . . .

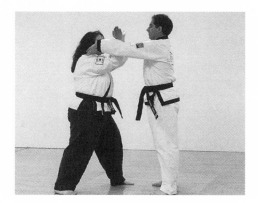

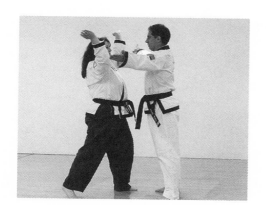

then when he releases his grip . . .

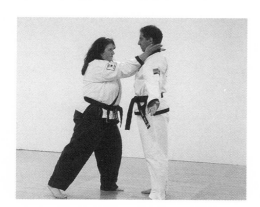

strike to his neck with both hands.

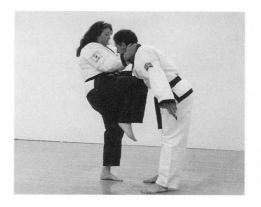

Finally, grab him behind the head and pull him down into a knee strike.

Self-Defense Against a Two-Handed Chokehold

When coked from the front, raise one arm up . . .

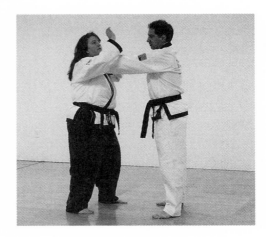

cross over the attacker's arms . . .

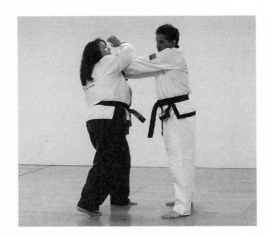

and execute an elbow strike to his head.

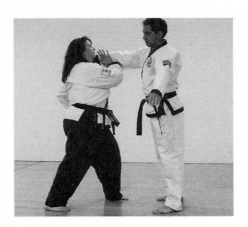

Self-Defense Against a Two-Handed Chokehold

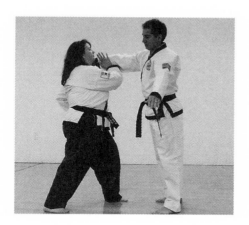

When choked from the front, push away your attacker's right arm with your right hand . . .

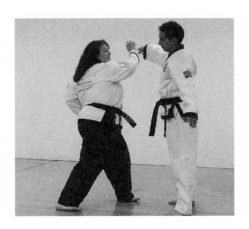

then do the same to his left arm with your left hand . . .

releasing his grip so you can escape.

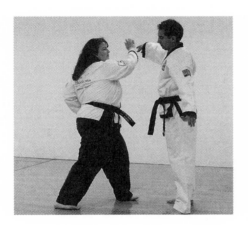

Self-Defense Against a Two-Handed Chokehold from Behind

When choked from behind, raise one arm . . .

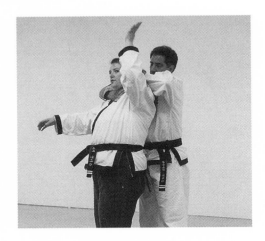

step and turn towards your upraised arm.

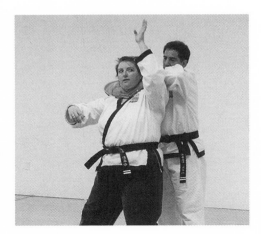

Keep turning until you break your attacker's grip.

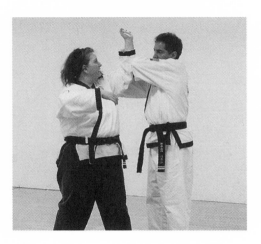

Self-Defense Against a Bearhug

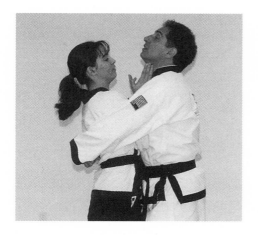

When grabbed over your arms, bring both hands up between youself and your attacker.

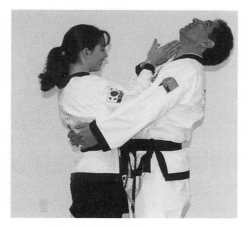

Press his throat away from you with your hands . . .

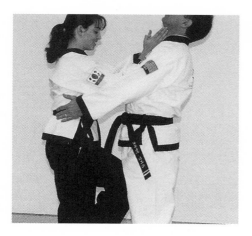

followed by a knee strike to the groin.

Self-Defense Against a Bearhug from Behind

When grabbed from behind . . .

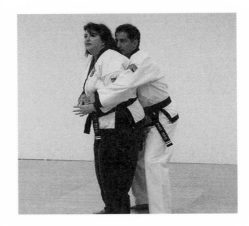

lean forward to unbalance the attacker.

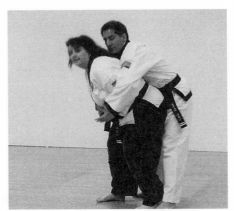

Quickly stand up and step to the side.

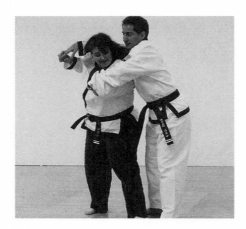

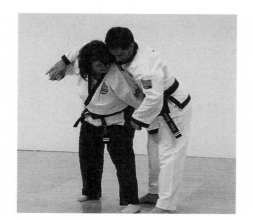

Strike to the groin.

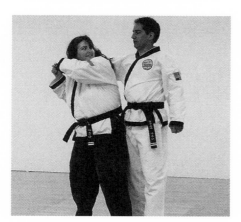

Then stand up quickly again . . .

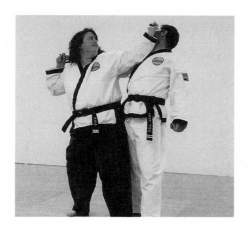

and strike to the face.

Self-Defense Against a Bearhug from Behind

When grabbed from behind with both arms trapped . . .

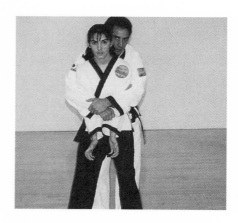

bend forward and grab one of your attacker's legs.

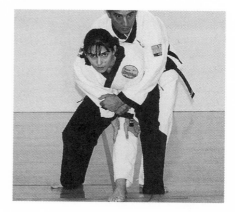

Pull his leg upward until he falls, allowing you to escape.

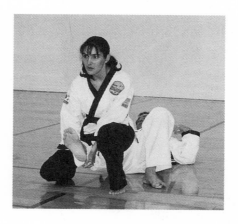

Self-Defense Against a Hair Grab

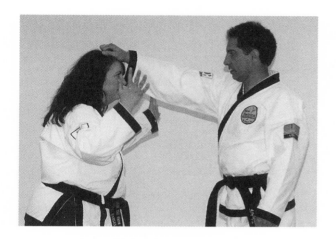

When grabbed by the hair . . .

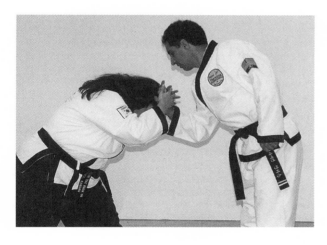

hold your attacker's hand firmly against your head with both hands and bend down.

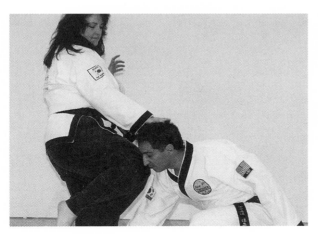

As your attacker falls, stand up quickly and strike his head with your knee.

Self-Defense Against a Full-Nelson Hold

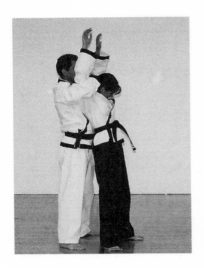

When grabbed in a full nelson, raise both arms.

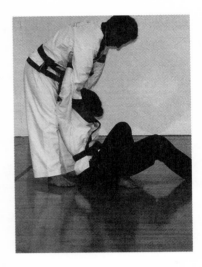

Relax your body and drop straight down to a seated position.

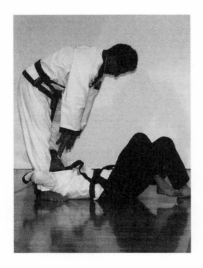

Grasp your attacker's ankles.

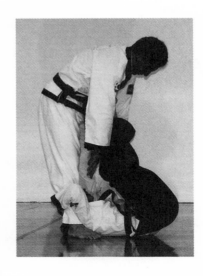

Kick to his stomach or face.

Self-Defense from a Seated Position

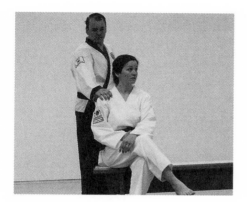

When grabbed from behind in a seated position . . .

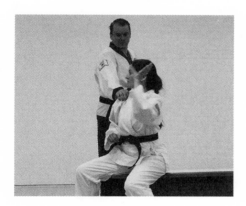

quickly turn around toward your attacker and perpare to strike.

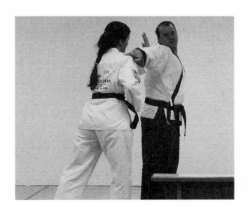

Stand up and strike to your attacker's elbow with your palm to break his grip.

Self-Defense from a Seated Position

When choked from behind, grasp your attacker's arm and pull him forward.

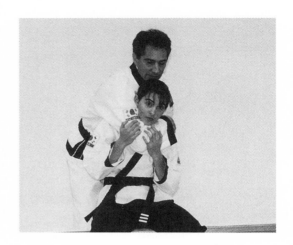

As he moves forward, grasp his shoulder and plant your feet firmly.

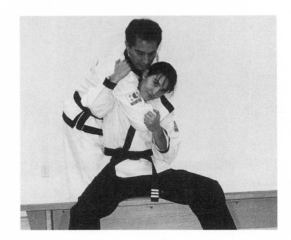

Pull him over the bench by leaning forward and turning.

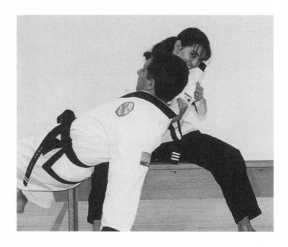

Self-Defense from the Ground

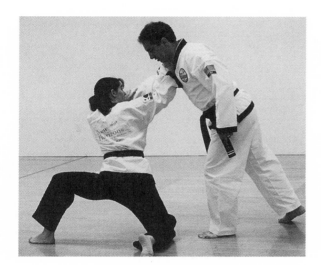

When grabbed in a kneeling position, grasp your attacker's wrist and shoulder . . .

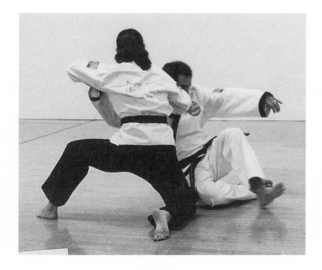

Turn away from the attacker, pulling him to the ground as you prepare to stand up.

Self-Defense from the Ground

When appraoched in a prone position, kick to the attacker's knee to knock him down . . .

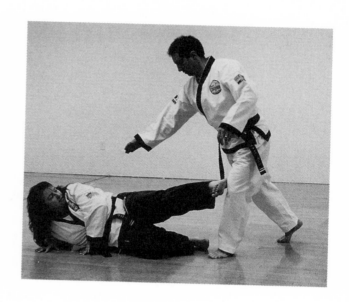

then kick to his ribs to stop his attack.

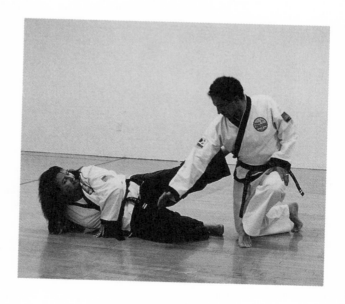

Self-Defense from the Ground

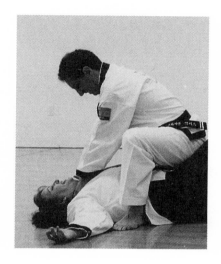

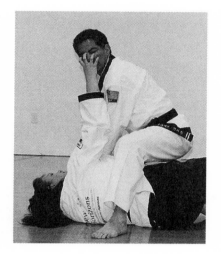

*When attacked
on the ground . . .*

strike to the attacker's eyes.

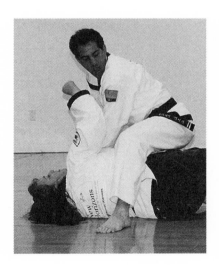

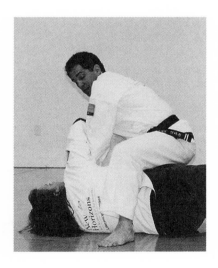

*Roll in the direction
of your stirke . . .*

*and throw him off,
allowing you to escape.*

5

Sparring

I'll be honest with you. I'm not sure what I'd do if I practiced a martial art that didn't include sparring—free style fighting. I don't think I'd last very long at it. This is not because I am so good at sparring or because it makes me feel I could beat up anybody—it is just that I've never participated in anything like it, and I've never reached a point where I say, there's not much more I can learn. Of course, I have the benefit of great partners and inspired instructors, so I'm probably at an advantage. Some people never learn to enjoy sparring, even though it is in integral part of most martial arts styles. I've noticed that many women get frustrated when they spar because much of what they are taught is based on male-oriented models. What works for men against each other does not necessarily work for a woman against a man.

Learning to see size difference as an advantage can improve one's sparring tremendously. For women, who have less body mass at their disposal than most men, power will be acquired by relying on speed more than mass.

First, though, some discussion about contact. Many schools expect little or no contact from their fighters. Others allow some contact; and still others are full contact. The most responsible schools that advocate contact sparring also insist on controlled contact. The point, after all, is to become good at sparring, not to injure your partner. But as long as there are black belts, and as long as some of them are men, no sparring among black belts will remain light and controlled. And your opinion of what is light contact and your partner's opinion of what is light contact may vary considerably. Keep in mind as well the bully factor; guys who wouldn't dare pick on someone their own size will whale away on smaller people. Now, I couldn't get away with smacking around kids half my size, but the fact that I'm half the size of the man I'm sparring seems to have no bearing on how hard he thinks he can go. He'll either patronize me (for which he'll get a nice sharp hooking kick to the side of the head) or he'll try to run me over. This is true even of the men who otherwise adore and worship the ground you walk on. They'll smack you with a spinning heel kick and when you pick yourself up they'll be all concern ("Are you okay? You're not mad at me? Oh, look at that bruise.") This won't prevent them from clocking you with that kick again should the opportunity present itself. Therefore: be ready for more contact than you might otherwise like. Also be prepared to insist that they back it down.

I have been known to zap someone pretty hard in a not quite target area if they won't back off, so that when they complain, I will point out that I had already asked them to back off and they hadn't. Sometimes you'll get a guy who thinks going full force against someone half his size is good for the person being attacked full force. The excuse is always, "Well, in a street fight you'd need to learn how to handle a bigger attacker." This is true. And one of the reasons we spar is so that we will be prepared to defend ourselves should we run into a bad man on the street. But point out to your partner that you are sparring, not brawling, and if he wants to make the groin a legal target, as it would be in a street fight, you'd like that. If he agrees you can go after his knees so that the practice is more "realistic," you'd be happy to do so. It is ridiculous to think of sparring as anything like a street fight, so don't let people tell you it is. Sparring helps you become a better martial artist, and it also helps you get used to being struck, and these are things that will help you in a street fight.

Wear protective gear—shin guards, forearm guards, hip pads and a chest protector. Most of these will fit under your uniform, and after some practice are very comfortable to wear. They'll pad some of the blows you receive and will make you less worried about getting hit. Your partner should protect him or herself in the same way. Padded gloves, footgear and headgear are recommended as well.

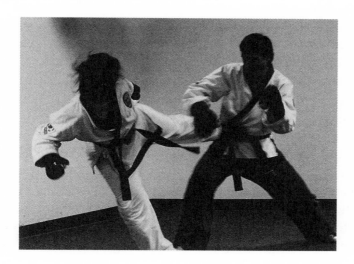

Finally, keep in mind that learning to take a tough kick does more than prepare you for a real confrontation. Shaking off that roundhouse kick while in the relative safety of the training hall may actually help you when you're knocked in the head outside the confines of the place—both literally and figuratively.

First off, you'll see I'm assuming you're sparring men as well as women. Women will teach you about speed, flexibility and technique, but really only men can weigh 250 and be mostly muscle, so it's important to spar them as well. Reconsider any school that routinely separates students along gender lines. (I work out with guys who are smaller than I am, so I've always thought it pretty stupid to assume size is automatically related to gender). Women-only classes can be great for morale and can encourage the free exchange of ideas and other benefits that might otherwise not exist, but it probably isn't a great idea to practice martial arts only with women. Men do have some insight as well. And when you make that 250 pound linebacker take a step back when you deliver a kick, it gives you some confidence in your skills and abilities. Again, however, training only with men will stunt your growth as a martial artist. It also puts you at a serious disadvantage should you wish to spar in tournaments.

Sparring Psychology

The first thing that men learn, when they are about six weeks old, is the foundation of sports psychology ("TEAM doesn't have any I in it!"). Women are busy being indoctrinated with other nonsense, so they are usually a little older before they are exposed to this stuff. But men do learn something about strategy and tactics from knocking each other around in mock wrestling contests and pseudo-football games. You ever play pick up basketball with a man? Can you say personal foul? If he can get away with it, it's okay. Men learn quickly that if they can rattle the opponent, that's half the battle. That's why guys talk trash. If you make someone mad, they're no longer in the game, they're focusing on you or what you said, which makes them more vulnerable to getting beaten. You and I might call this stuff cheating, but they call it psyching the opponent out, or getting them out of their game. When it is time for the kicker to kick the game-winning field goal, the opposing team will call a time out just as the kicker is about to put his toe to the cowhide. This means his mental focus will be challenged, shaken up. It also means that every time he lines up to kick the ball, he's wondering, are they going to call a time out or not? This silliness is considered an important part of the psychology of football, called icing the kicker. Personally, I think when a game hinges on your having to psych out the other team's field goal kicker, it is time for you to get a brand new offensive line.

Another example: the players from both football teams who are lined up on the line of scrimmage have to remain still until the ball is snapped to the quarterback (yes, this is the simplistic version). If any player who is lined up on the line of scrimmage moves before the ball is snapped to the quarterback, their team gets penalized. The purpose of this rule is to keep things fair until the play actually starts. Everyone therefore gets a fair shot at either making a play or stopping a play. Depending on what side of the ball you are on, moving before the ball is snapped is either a false start or an offsides call. Unless you are a football addict, you would not believe the amount of effort that goes into trying to make the other team move before they are supposed to.

To get drawn offsides is like getting suckered; the opposing linemen will shake their heads saying, I can't believe you fell for it. Some NFL guys are known in the league for being able to flinch ever so perfectly, just enough so that they won't get a penalty for moving, but enough to make the other team think the play has started and to make them move forward. Linemen actually work on this flinch. They admire the finesse with which grown men flex muscles at each other in an attempt to make the other side move first. Then they all get excited and hug each other. Teams who get mad when this happens to them are a source of great amusement. Players who can draw other teams offsides without getting into trouble themselves are greatly admired. This is considered a very cool trait. It is thought to get the other side out of their game, psyching them out with what you and I would call cheating, because it violates the spirit of the law if not the letter of it. But men think it is a very worthy endeavor. Therefore, guys are forever trying to act like football players and get you out of your game. If they do, they feel they have won some sort of contest, and the most frustrating thing for us is that we don't even know a contest is going on half the time.

It is true that the person who controls the energy and momentum of a match will have a good chance of winning it, and when you spar according to what works best for you, you are more likely to win. But men will go to bizarre and crazy lengths to get you out of your game, even if you manage to chew 'em up and spit 'em out otherwise.

In sparring, a match starts when the judge or instructors says "go," and the two contestants signal their intention to fight by kihoping or shouting. I've sparred one man who shouts and kicks at the same time, thinking the split second difference makes him a winner. All the other guys think this is a great strategy. All the women think this is cheating (you're supposed to wait until *after* you kihop to begin sparring). You cannot reason with a person like this. You must simply know what he is going to do and then avoid the kick.

Another set of rules describes the target area. All techniques must be above the opponent's waist. The back is not a legal target area, nor is the back of the head. Therefore, most women try not to hit their partners in non-target areas. If they accidentally make contact with someone in a non-contact area, they will apologize. But men, on the other hand, think a non-target area is simply an area that doesn't count toward a point total. Some will routinely strike to non-target areas much as a boxer might jab, simply to see what the response will be. He knows that even if he does make contact, it doesn't count as a point, but he doesn't see that trying to make contact to a non-target area is wrong. He'll continually kick to your hip, for instance, even though he won't score any points for it, even though it is not a target area, and he'll do this just to get you out of your game. One person I have sparred with frequently uses this technique all the time. He'll kick to the hip all the time. I've watched people (not just women) stop the sparring to tell him to get his kicks up. He ignores this, just nodding and smiling. Then he continues to kick to the hip. Then, if his partner gets frustrated or angry, he or she won't spar as well. And this man thinks he has won because he got his opponent out of his or her game by kicking to an illegal target area. As you may have guessed, this angers the women and pleases the men. Perhaps we should start jabbing to the groin to get them out of their game.

However, the mental and emotional aspects of a sparring match should not be overlooked. It is important to stay focused and not be distracted by irrelevant, nonessential things going on around you. If you don't let them provoke you out of your game, after a while they'll quit trying.

The best thing I learned was never to worry about what the other guy is doing. I concern myself only with the number of points I score on my opponent, not the number he scores on me. This has helped my focus tremendously and also keeps me from falling victim to the little games others might play. Look your partner in the eye and go after him.

As discussed in Chapter Two, certain guys at certain ages and at certain ranks develop an attitude problem toward women, thinking they aren't as challenging or rewarding to spar as men. This attitude is fed by martial arts publications that ask "Should women be in the training hall?" (the actual title of an article I saw in a martial arts magazine that I once respected.) These kinds of rhetorical questions are frustrating because they assume that men are the legitimate martial artists and women are only a distraction at best and poor competition regardless. My question is, why should men be allowed in the training hall? In this day and age, to be able to ask such ridiculous questions is beyond my comprehension. Still, it does affect us and that's why it's important to judge a school by its commitment to discouraging gender stereotyping. Still, as in all endeavors, the best way to defeat ridiculous attitudes is by defeating the idiots who have them, which is always a pleasure anyway.

The true competition is against yourself. This is why you should focus on what you do. Did you counter that strike or was your timing off? Did you just block when you could have countered? Did you keep pushing him back or did you quit going after him once you executed two techniques in a row?

As usual, discussions with your partners can be immensely helpful. If possible, arrange to spar someone who'll be willing to stop in the middle of the match and point out what you could have done or what you should have done—or what you did do! (Praise is also good). Videotaping sparring matches can be very enlightening, although it can be difficult to see beyond the "I can't believe I look like that" stage. If you watch your sparring matches on video, you'll count the number of openings you had and missed and you'll want to kick yourself, but it will help you learn what your strengths are and what your major weaknesses might be. Sometimes, fixing one weakness will eliminate others as well. If you put too much weight on your back leg, for instance, not only will you have difficulty doing reverse kicks and the like, but your ability to evade the opponent by footwork will be limited. If you're too upright, you'll have difficulty increasing your speed, and you'll have problems with balance, so that every technique you do will be off-balance and off-target. Quick corrections can make major changes in your skill level.

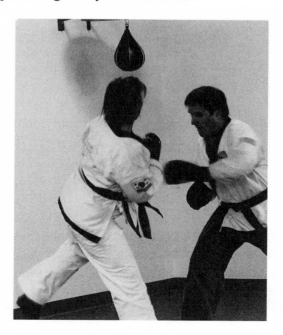

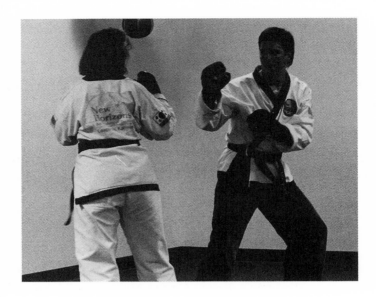

Sizing Up Your Opponent

Watch how you spar different kinds of people. Do you spar tall people the same way you spar short ones? Do you spar heavy contact fighters the same way you spar light contact fighters? You shouldn't. If one opponent relies on a fast-paced, aggressive attack, your approach should be different from what you do when you face a fighter who relies primarily on defensive countering techniques. This is not to say that your opponent should dictate the match, or that you can't rely on certain techniques and sequences that work well for you, just that you should respond to each individual as just that—a different individual. If one person never gets out of the way of your ax kick, by all means use it every chance you get. If another person easily evades it and lands a spinning heel kick on your head whenever your try, a new tactic is called for. This also means you'll add variety to your sparring.

Since I'm short, I relied a lot on punches for years, even practicing boxing to improve my punching skills. I had a good front kick that I'd use to kick to the mid-section, and a good roundhouse kick that I'd use to kick high. I would use these kicks in order to get into punching range. Then I'd use the front kick to push back out of punching range. It worked for me until I met a fighter who'd go inside before I could get there and would jam up all my techniques. I had to add a sidekick to keep him outside, and then I added a reverse kick for the times when a sidekick didn't keep him outside. I'd just launch the reverse kick to give me a chance to move outside and set things up my way. These techniques worked well—and continue to work well for me.

When I first added these techniques to my arsenal, the people I spar on a regular basis found me much harder than usual to spar—not because the techniques were so advanced or so difficult to defend against or counter— just because they were not techniques I normally used. This convinced me that to remain unpredictable, I needed to be adding new kicks and punches and new combinations of them to my arsenal all the time. By the same token, I take out things that I have done over and over. For instance, many times the people I spar assume I am setting up to do an ax kick. But since everyone knows that I set up to do ax kicks a certain way, I no longer use ax kicks, or at least not very much. Everyone got wise to it and learned to read it coming from a mile off. Thus, you need to switch things into and out of your sparring arsenal. When people quit expecting my ax kick, that's when I'll start using it again.

Responding differently to each individual partner helps you to do this, to vary your routine and add what works and subtract what doesn't. Your sparring should be a work in progress, not a final product. That way, it can change as you do, grow as you learn, mature as you do, and adjust to the changes in your skill level, and physical ability. Instead of simply thinking, "I am not doing so well with this kind of fighter, no big deal, I do great everywhere else," find out what you can do to defeat this more challenging opponent.

One of the great things I do is people-watch. Since I began practicing martial arts, I have taken this a step further. As I walk down the street, I think of the different techniques that might work on the different people I see. Not only does this make me see the wide variety of people in the world, and discourage me from relying too much on one or two basic techniques, it also helps me feel confident that I could respond to a threat more appropriately and more immediately than if I never bothered to be aware of the people around me.

In addition, I observe as much martial arts practice as I can. For instance, I watched at a regional tournament as year after year a certain woman always won her women's sparring division, and would go on to win the women's grand champion trophy. She relied on a back leg roundhouse kick, which is Olympic-style Tae Kwon Do, while most of the women she fought practiced traditional-style Tae Kwon Do. Now traditional-style Tae Kwon Do will beat Olympic style every time (plus it's a lot more fun to watch) but you have to be incredibly fast. Those of us who watched and who practiced traditional-style kept saying, "She leaves herself wide open every time she does that kick. If only someone would throw a reverse kick." Of course, the champion was very quick. Although she was open when she kicked, she didn't stay open long—and her kicks were so powerful that no one wanted to turn their backs on them. But one woman who got tired of being defeated for grand champion practiced reverse kicks until she could do them so quickly you could barely see them—but you could sure feel them. And she absolutely devastated the former champion, who'd relied on that roundhouse kick for so long, even though its inherent weakness was obvious to everyone, that she simply had nothing else to come back with.

So mix it up, let it evolve, learn from watching others. This observation is also of greater benefit if you ask why they do what they do. Explain what you saw (I noticed you always counter a reverse kick with a reverse punch. Why?). And when you are impressed by a fighter, and by all means let yourself be impressed by a fighter, think not only about what works and why, but also think about alternatives that would work equally well, say a reverse kick instead of a reverse punch. And then think of the different ways to defeat the techniques you've seen. If you do a reverse kick and your partner evades and scores with a reverse punch, what can you do to prevent her from using that reverse punch effectively, other than never using your reverse kick again? Maybe two quick reverse kicks in a row would work. Try it out with a partner. Practice until you get a feel for the sequence, then try it sparring. Don't give up after just one try. It's okay to make mistakes and be slow. Nothing works as perfectly as you'd like the first time. Only if it clearly has no hope of working should you abandon it. The practice and implementation of new techniques is difficult—it's easier and far more comfortable to rely on the same old techniques we've already mastered and are comfortable with. But like my ax kick, these grow predictable over time. You don't continue to grow as a martial artist without challenging yourself. And some of your techniques that once worked effectively no longer do so because your partners have thought their way past them as well. So continually expanding and changing your repertoire is healthy and desirable. Your sparring is always a work in progress and you should learn constantly from it.

Finding Your Strengths

If you don't care much for sparring, it's hard to imagine devoting the time necessary to make improvements. Many people dislike sparring because they aren't very good at it. This is probably the primary reason women don't like sparring (though probably 90% of all female martial artists I know list sparring as their favorite part of martial arts practice). Some women are afraid of hurting themselves or someone else. But it is primarily a lack of confidence that leads to a dislike of the sport. If you don't do well in sparring, you won't want to spar and then you won't spar well, you'll simply be trying to get it all over with, so there will be little room for improvement or for taking pleasure in the activity.

As I have said, sparring is my favorite part of class, but it wasn't always so. When I think back to my early days, I remember that I used to attend certain classes that were designated non-sparring classes. We worked on specific self-defense techniques in these classes instead of on free-style fighting. These classes were held at the beginning of the week and I looked forward to them because I would not have to spar. Since I found physical contact very unnerving, it doesn't surprise me that sparring was not my favorite way to spend time. What surprises me is how quickly I learned to love it and how soon it did become my favorite part of class.

I liked the way it presented new and fresh challenges every day. Some people prefer to work on the areas over which they have more control— body conditioning, forms, and the like. These require only one person, you can do it pretty easily anywhere, and you're not actually competing with anyone (except yourself). There isn't always a winner or loser. I don't think in those terms, however. Regardless of who does what during the sparring match, I always feel like a winner regardless of how many points my opponent scored on me. If I learned something, tried something new, included a technique I have been working on, or just plain performed better than usual, I am happy. I feel as if I am taking something rewarding and valuable away from the encounter.

As you think about improving your sparring, remember that the more you practice, the more confident you will be and the more you will like sparring. I don't guarantee you'll ever love it, but if you practice timing techniques with a partner at least five minutes every day, I do guarantee that you'll be smarter and wiser in the ring and you probably will enjoy the experience more than you otherwise would. Remember that until you reach a certain minimum level of competence in sparring, it is difficult to enjoy. You feel nervous, you lack confidence, you are unsure. Once you become a little better, you can relax and enjoy the process more.

Consider yourself. Take an honest inventory of your body type. A physical therapist once told me that short stocky people like me could do well in martial arts because our tendons, ligaments and muscles responded more quickly with less trauma to the techniques than did tall, lanky people with long muscles, tendons and ligaments. My experience has been that I do suffer fewer sprains and strains than the tall people do, but this is the only advantage I have over them. I am, however, a lot faster than I look, which still continues to amaze and annoy my sparring partners. If I take stock, I see I am shorter than most of the people I work out with, and while I am lighter than almost all of the men, I am heavier than about half of the women. This means that in an exchange of kicks, the taller person, who is almost everyone else in the school, has the advantage over me. The reach of a tall person is longer. So I have to make sure that other ranges are used. Since I am heavier than some of the women, I probably won't beat them with my speed, though as I said I am faster than I look. Therefore, if we exchange kicks, I will be at a disadvantage because mine won't be so fast. I am more flexible than most of the guys, but still I can't kick a 6 foot guy in the head all that easily, because I am pretty short. This gives me a little advantage, however, over people who are nearer me in height and aren't as flexible. I actually have more target area to score on because of my flexibility, whereas a less flexible person actually has less area to score on.

After assessing my build and comparing it with the people I work out with, it is easy for me to see why I like fighting in close. It makes the tall guys nervous. Once out of kicking range, they don't know quite what to do. It also concerns the women who like to counter defensively; once inside they run out of counters to use, especially since they rely primarily on kicks as counters, and we are not in kicking range. When nose to nose, just how do you counter an uppercut? All you can really do is trade blows, but because I have been doing this forever, and because I'm quick, I can get in there, land a punch and get out again. So being short has compensatory factors. Also, my speed is less important when punching, since these are much more direct and quicker to reach the target than kicks are. Therefore, I have found a style that suits me well.

However, my greatest weakness occurs at the moment when I attempt to make the move from kicking range to punching range. If I am going to get nailed, it is right when I make this transition. And while I try to camouflage what I am doing, anyone who has sparred me more than once knows that I am going to try to go inside. The moving back outside is usually uneventful because my partner is usually glad that I am moving to a more civilized range, and he or she won't try to stop me.

So I know when I am most vulnerable. I also know what techniques stop me cold. A sidekick to the ribs, for instance, will stop me every time, even when other techniques don't even slow me down. I have felt more feet planted in my rib cage than in any other target area on my body. I continue to get sterling advice like, "cover up when you go in," but that is easy for the person who is kicking me to say. So I learned to distract my partners while I moved in. I would fake a kick high and then slide forward and punch to the middle. This worked well except on a 6 foot guy who would laugh at my attempts to go high. If I tried to use a kick to enter, this partner would simply back up a step. So I learned a lunge kick that covered a lot of territory, so that even if this partner took a step back, I would still tag him with the kick and be able to move into fighting range. I learned that feinting high, then moving in, punching to the middle and moving out with a middle front kick worked well routinely. I have to add variety to this and change it all the time; sometimes I use a hooking kick high, and sometimes a spinning backfist, but the sequence is the same—high, middle, middle, out. Sometimes I spar people who are really good inside, which is hard for me. You'd think since I love to do it, I would have thought of ways to counter me before now, but no such luck. I am still as puzzled by people coming inside on me as they are when I come inside on them. Mostly I move back to kicking range using one of a variety of bail-out techniques, such as a tightly chambered reverse kick, a middle front kick, or a spinning backfist. I also use footwork to sidestep someone inside, then punch to the ribs and work my way outside.

Consider your height, size, principal techniques and sparring goals. Do you want to hit 6 foot guys in the head with a round house kick? Then certain steps should be taken to ensure flexibility, and to ensure good technique, both of which, along with good balance, contribute to the ability to reach high with your kicks.

Conditioning for Sparring

Flexibility training is most helpful, and women are actually more likely to make significant gains in flexibility than men. Remember if you do any weight training that the more muscle bulk you build up, the less flexibility you retain. Therefore, people who are building muscle mass must work especially hard to remain flexible and improve their flexibility. Always warming up and stretching before class and then cooling down and stretching afterward will help you become more flexible, as well as help prevent injuries. Keep in mind that additional stretching can be done any time throughout the day. People who work at desks for long periods of time know that pausing to stretch neck, shoulder and arms throughout the course of the day can prevent painful muscle tension and subsequent headaches and yet they often don't go a step further—stretching hips, knees and ankles. This can be done in the restroom if you don't have privacy at work. Stretch at other times throughout the day. Read the newspaper on the floor while doing an open stretch. I know a school teacher who grades papers this way, students who study this way and workers who watch T.V. this way. Stretching whenever possible helps to improve and maintain your flexibility.

In addition, speed can be increased a number of ways. Perhaps the best way is to fuel your body appropriately. The better you eat, the more energy you have, the more you are able to feel you can tackle anything. Consider. Those days when you have eaten too much of the wrong kind of food—you feel slow and bloated. In fact, most of us are in such a hurry that our nutrition is so poor it is a wonder we have the energy to do anything.

Eat right, get your rest—easy to say, I know, harder to do, but the quickest way to become a better competitor is to treat your body with kindness and respect. Forget artificial stimulants like caffeine. With proper rest and nutrition you'll have so much energy, you won't need that cup of coffee or that candy bar to give you a boost. And after a while, you will prefer fruit and veggies to chips and ice cream. So a sensible eating plan, a better managed schedule and at least 8 hours sleep are the places to start, because without them, you will never get anywhere.

Add some flexibility training and you are on your way. Other methods for increasing speed include plyometrics. This is the art of building up the short twitch muscle fibers—the quick burst muscle fibers as opposed to the longer muscle fibers that are meant for endurance. Just compare a sprinter's legs to a marathoner's legs. Sprinters are stockier, shorter, more compact and their legs are huge. Marathoners on the other hand are tall and lanky—wiry, even. Their legs are long and lean. Both kinds of athletes are focusing on different sets of muscle fibers in their training. These two types of runners have overexaggerated certain muscle tendencies.

Far too many of us, however, don't work out our quick muscle fibers. Our workouts are aerobic, geared toward increasing our heart rate, improving our endurance, and expanding our lung capacity. These are great goals, because you want to be fit, healthy and active for a long time. But some attention should be paid to developing quickness. As in any attempt to build muscle, you must be persistent over time, but some improvement will be seen almost immediately.

Practice plyometric exercises, which are designed to give you explosive power. Frog jumps are a good example. Squatting on the floor, hands out in front for balance, leap frog your way across the room as quickly as possible. Your muscles will be burning before you know it. Try these once or twice a day, building up to ten repetitions twice a day. Other possibilities abound. The games you play with kids are great. Hopscotch, jump rope, you name it. All require balance, quickness, and timing, all of which are essential to good sparring skills.

For timing, half speed sparring is an excellent way to practice techniques. Also practicing on a speed bag like boxers do will help you with your timing. Any boxing instruction or boxing workout will help you understand the purpose of feints and jabs and the necessity of combining techniques together for maximum effect. This is an area where women can excel, since they can be faster than men. Frequently I watch sparring matches in which first one partner kicks and then the other partner kicks. Then the first partner blocks and counters, and then the second blocks and counters. While rhythm in sparring is sometimes desirable, especially when you are working on timing, you always want to think about persistence, about breaking up that rhythm, which creates unpredictability. If the first technique you use doesn't get through your partner's defense, maybe your second or third—or fourth—attempt will.

The value of practicing like this is it helps you visualize what might happen if you do meet an assailant on the street. Remember, you don't want to make him mad. You want to escape. So if your first punch doesn't do it, you don't want to just drop back in surprise and let him attack the perfect opening you've left for him. A continuous attack will disorient anyone, providing you with a possible opportunity to escape or you may disable your opponent enough to reduce the personal threat to you.

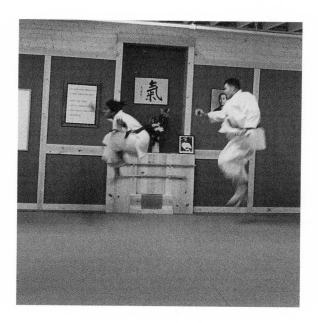

Plyometric exericses are an excellent method of improving your conditioning for sparring.

So vary the back-and-forth routine so common among martial artists by adding short bursts of speed and quick combinations of kicks and punches. Also, practicing your kicks against heavy targets or focus mitts will help you learn timing, improve your technique and judge your control.

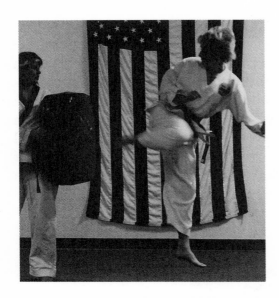

Use of a shield target is a good way to build power and speed in your kicks.

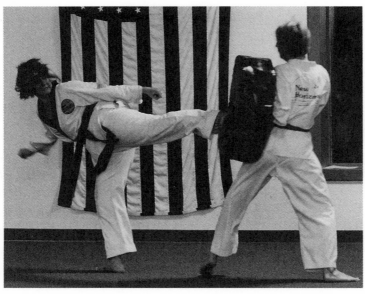

Finding Your Sparring Style

Continuous sparring for two-minute rounds is an excellent way to build up your endurance. It also helps you determine what combinations of techniques are most effective. Most people, sooner or later, develop a characteristic sparring style, and so should you. Don't let people tell you you're doing it all wrong and that you should spar just like they do. A person who prefers to spar defensively has just as much opportunity to win (a tournament, a brawl) as someone who wades in there aggressively and really goes after the opponent. Yes, the more aggressive person might be spectacular to watch and might seem to take control of a match early, but such a person can be beaten by his or her own aggressiveness—just standing back and waiting for the opening that will surely come is a tried and true method of handling aggressive fighters. But the same goes for the defensive method. It may be that the aggressive style will defeat the defensive style because the aggressive style fighter simply runs over the defensive fighter and wins before the defensive fighter has the opportunity to counter. Or it may be the defensive fighter exploits the weaknesses of the aggressive fighter before the aggressive fighter has gotten anywhere. So don't let anyone tell you that one kind of fighting is better than another. It depends on you, and to a lesser extent, on your opponent. But this does not mean that you shouldn't try new techniques and new combinations and new approaches as people suggest them to you or as you learn about them. Trying a variety of methods helps you select the approach and basic techniques you'll use in varying degrees throughout the rest of your sparring and martial arts career.

Identifying your style helps you capitalize on your strengths, but you should never dismiss suggestions and ideas immediately, without at least considering them, how they might apply, or how they could be adopted to suit your needs. What it does mean though, is that you should have confidence in your style and not change it because someone considers it a bit unusual. For instance, when I first started sparring, people discouraged me from going inside because I got kicked a lot as I would try to get into punching range. They thought I should spar in kicking range. But I am short and to make matters worse, my torso is long compared to my legs. So I am a short person with short legs. This means I will never win fighting in someone else's kicking range. What it means is that my kicking range is closer than anyone else's and it leads naturally to going into close range. It was not a bad style or poorly chosen techniques that made it difficult for me to capitalize on my in-close fighting preference, it was simply lack of experience, which plagues all beginning martial artists. People would actually make me stop what I was doing and go back to kicking range because they thought I would do better there. The problem was not with me. The problem was with my partners who were more comfortable sparring at kicking range. When I moved in, they might try to use a sidekick to keep me out of range, but if that didn't work, they had no idea what to do against me—they had no inside game. They would get flustered and irritated. I was getting them out of their game. (It was great.) My head instructor encouraged my style of fighting because he saw that it worked for me, and he got a kick out of the frustration it gave other fighters.

As I stuck with the style, some of my partners—those who could fight inside themselves—would help me out, and assisted me in improving and polishing my technique. Today no on tries to help me out by giving me pointers on staying in kicking range. Those who used to try to make me better now spend their time trying to make sure I don't get inside. If they can keep me out, they'll do okay, but they know that once I am inside, they don't have a chance. So instead of concentrating their efforts only on keeping me outside, they should also learn some techniques for handling me when I am inside, and some of them have—some of them have even learned the techniques from me! Because Tae Kwon Do is primarily a kicking art, it never occurred to many people how effective it can be fighting inside, because Tae Kwon Do has a lot of hand techniques, too. Not only that, though, the kicks can be used to maneuver you both into punching range and out of punching range without leaving you open. To simply walk into punching range is begging to get a foot in your chest. So you have to kick your way in; I usually jab a kick and instead of coming back to where I was, I let my foot drop right in front of my partner, then slide in with a punch or series of punches. The first kick covers me as I move in and distracts my partner, allowing me to punch. Then I will kick out with my back leg, before my opponent has a chance to start trading punches with me.

My sparring partners also found it unusual for a woman to punch so much (most women rely on kicks, particularly since women tend to have much more powerful lower bodies than upper bodies.) So they thought it was a bad idea for me to rely on punches. Also, since Tae Kwon Do has a great emphasis on kicking, they thought I was somehow not being true to the nature of the art. It was simply that they didn't expect women to punch and didn't know how to react. Once they became used to it, they realized that while it was true my legs were stronger than my arms, the advantage of using my size more than outweighed any differences in power. In fact, many of us learned together a great deal about fighting ranges, how they work, how to transition from one to another and how to use footwork without giving away your intentions. Just because I was stubborn. There are still people that I've been sparring for years and when I get inside they get frustrated and lose their focus. But they no longer doubt that I am doing a legitimate, intelligent thing. They just wish that they could prevent it.

Many styles allow a little contact to the head using kicks and limited hand techniques. Just as getting in close to punch the body is a great technique for women, so too are hand techniques to the head. In my school, the only hand technique to the head that we use are backfists, since they are less dangerous than straight punches, though we occasionally throw punches, knife hands and ridge hands when black belts spar each other.

These hand techniques are great because you can go high when you are in close and get your partner to raise his hands to block, thus exposing the middle. This is a great way to access two different target areas—high and middle—from the inside. Then, as your partner backs away or spins out of range, you can follow with a high or middle foot technique, causing uncertainty and confusion.

Developing Power

One of my many frustrations as a beginning martial artist was when I would kick someone during sparring, usually someone who was a lot bigger than I was, and I would basically bounce off them. The energy of my technique was being rebounded toward me. This is an odd happening that occurs when people throw themselves at otherwise immoveable objects. I learned that it was worth having happen because I would sure hate to get in a fight on the street and find that all my kicks were doing was causing me to bounce off my attacker. The best way to prevent this recoiling of energy (which is a problem not limited to women, but since we are smaller, it does happen to us more) is not necessarily to become stronger or more powerful, although this does help, but instead to develop a better understanding of the movement of energy so that you can transfer your energy to the target of your choice, instead of absorbing the energy yourself. To learn the balance and transfer of energy, you need to understand the difference between practice kicking (when you are kicking air), controlled kicking, and full contact kicking.

When you practice your kicks—perhaps in line during class—your target is imaginary. Nothing absorbs your energy, so if you kick too hard, you could hyperextend your knee or your hip. The reason is simple— it is your joint that ends up absorbing all that otherwise undissipated energy. Once it has been unleashed, it has to be transferred, absorbed or otherwise accounted for. When you kick correctly during line kicking, the energy you use to swing your leg forward becomes the momentum that brings your leg back to the starting position. But if you use too much energy, when your leg stops, your joint keeps going, instead of stopping as well and then swinging back down. You probably do want your kicks to snap or whip but not so that you do damage to yourself. Therefore, line kicking is a good time to work on technique and speed, not so much power. The control and focus required to achieve perfect technique on each kick won't allow lots of excess energy to be floating around, so you are less likely to hurt yourself. Remember that power comes from speed and mass, so working on speed will improve your power. When you are kicking for speed, the amount of energy needed to keep the leg moving forward and back absorbs the energy of the kick.

When you do controlled kicking, such as during sparring, or other practice with a focus mitt or pad, some of your energy is being absorbed by the target itself. So your quick kick, since it makes contact with a human or a pad, is slowed down markedly. Thus, you lose a little momentum; this means your kick is faster on the way to the target than it is on the way back from the target. Controlled sparring is a good way to practice speed because it is very difficult to control very quick kicks, which by the nature of their speed can be quite powerful.

Assume you're working on technique and you are sparring at half speed to be certain each movement is correct. If each movement consists of an equivalent amount of energy, your body will allow for it and you won't fall on your head or bounce off your target. But let's say you are doing a sidekick slowly for technique. You chamber high, push it out, pivot on your supporting foot, all the while your body is making the minute adjustments necessary for you to maintain your balance. But if one part of your kick was suddenly performed at a different speed, or used a different amount of energy, you'd find yourself in trouble. Say you suddenly snap the last bit of that slow sidekick out. The sudden change in energy will probably cause you to lose balance—until you have trained for it. You may not fall, but you will certainly feel your body making sudden major adjustments.

Controlled kicking then requires a redistribution of energy in the form of balance and control. If any of these is weak, the energy becomes loose, in a manner of speaking, and you lose control or mastery over your body and your kick, and you may fall, or you may strike the target harder than you intended.

When you do a kick full power, especially before you have practiced the technique a great deal, your body can't account for the sudden energy very quickly, so it recoils back on you and you bounce. That's why you need practice doing full contact techniques. You'll learn to control the kick, redistribute your weight and maintain your balance all while focusing your energy on the target, which if the technique is done correctly, will absorb all the energy. Or in the case of boards and people, will absorb all the damage. But these elements don't come easy, so you have to practice full contact. Since relatively few martial artists care to spar full contact, and because it is dangerous to kick air full contact, you should invest in a heavy bag. Heavily padded targets are good for training for power and focus, but often full contact kicking is still too hard for these targets to absorb all the power; some of it will get transferred to the target holder.

Working with targets helps you go full speed with controlled power and learn if you are landing your technique correctly all the time. You are able to feel when your kick is too high or too low or off center. Your partner can also comment on what he or she sees and feels; the stronger kicks are more noticeable; the better techniques are easily identified. Since you can use more power than you ordinarily would in sparring, target kicking can help you being to learn to kick without bouncing off the target. But heavy bag training is an absolute necessity to learn how to do this. A heavy bag is like a person; it is heavy and more solid than it looks. You can kick it pretty hard and it won't move, just like some people.

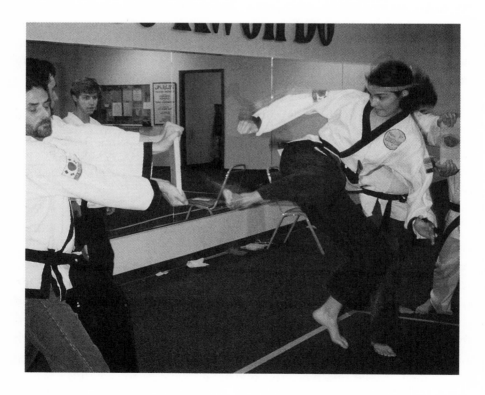

Board breaking is a method of testing the power of kicks and strikes.

Unlike a partner, who might be encouraging you or who may be a little less than honest, the heavy bag never lies. If you are off target, you'll know it. If you are too high or too low, you'll know it. You'll probably fall down, which is how you will know it. The heavy bag doesn't move with your kick the way a sparring partner does. It just hangs there. If you hit it hard, you might bounce off. So you must learn how to keep yourself solid while you are kicking. To kick the heavy bag so that the blow is powerful enough to move it instead of you, you must hit it accurately, and you must hit it hard, transferring your energy to it. Once you've gotten the idea of hitting the heavy bag, you can work on doing all your techniques full power, making corrections in balance and technique as you find yourself bouncing off it. If you master this, you will rarely find yourself bouncing off partners during sparring.

In some styles, board breaking is part of the art. In those styles, a similar set of principles apply. If you don't do the technique correctly, with speed and power, you will simply bounce off the board. While bouncing off an opponent in a sparring match feels foolish, it usually hurts nothing but your pride. Bouncing off boards is another matter entirely. Breaking a board is simply a matter of correctly transferring your energy to the board, where the board cannot absorb the power adequately and so breaks from the force of the blow.

Sparring is definitely a mental game. Controlling your emotions and learning to focus are key to becoming an excellent fighter. But techniques also need to be developed and perfected. The next chapter will describe these briefly.

6

Techniques

The purpose of this chapter is to help you identify those techniques that work best for you, and to understand why other techniques are more difficult to execute well. Understanding why can help you succeed. But one caveat: every single martial arts technique can be mastered by a woman. It is just that some techniques require more patience and training for women to master; others, such as those that rely on speed or flexibility, usually require less patience and time. The techniques of most martial arts were created by and for men, and since women are built differently, we sometimes find certain techniques problematic to execute. This is not to say that some men don't find the same techniques difficult; nor does it mean that all women find the same techniques difficult. The point of this chapter is simply to help you master techniques that give people trouble, and to use your strengths to their best advantage.

Jumping Kicks

One example of a technique that often gives women trouble is the jumping kick. I have seen plenty of women perform high jumping kicks flawlessly from the time they are first introduced to them. But I was never one of those women, and I know quite a number of women who weren't either. Jumping kicks always required much practice and training for me. The first problem, of course, is my hips—the fact that I have them. This makes my center of gravity lower than a man's, which means it requires more skill and effort for me to jump and execute a kicking technique. In this case, it is a simple matter of body structure. Spinning in the air and leaping about is not exactly a natural state of being for an individual with a womanly figure. Nor, truth be told, is it a natural state for men with beer bellies, but they do have the advantage of a different, more forgiving, body structure.

The best way to improve jumping techniques is to separate the technique into its various parts. For instance, a jump front kick can be broken into the jump and the front kick itself. Practice jumping first without worrying about the front kick. Try to jump as high as you can while still maintaining your balance. Then put the jump and the kick together. Each jumping technique requires a slightly different kind of jump, so each jump should be practiced separately. For a jump reverse sidekick, unlike a jump front kick, you must rotate while in the air. This is a much different technique from the jump front kick, where you simply jump as high as you can, then perform the kick to the front or forward position. For a jump reverse sidekick, try jumping and tucking your legs under you so that your calves touch your thighs. This helps you gain more height and also puts your legs in a better position to execute the kick. Once you can do this successfully, try spinning in the air as you jump and tuck your legs. Then, when you are comfortable with this, you can add the reverse sidekick.

Plyometric drills are helpful in improving your ability to perform jumping kicks. Plyometrics help you gain explosive power and explosive movements. Such exercises can help in areas other than jumping techniques; they improve quickness and response time as well. One simple drill is to stack a few kicking targets on the floor and jump from one side to the others, as quickly as you can, without pausing between jumps and without knocking the targets over. Stack the targets higher as you improve. Another good drill is to have a partner, using a target or focus mitt, sweep at your feet so that you must jump up to avoid being hit by the target. Your partner should work quickly, not allowing pauses between jumps. One note—always use soft materials such as kicking targets for these drills. Using a chair or bench to jump over can be dangerous if you miss or if you catch your foot.

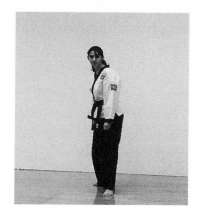

One method of developing jumping kicks is to practice jumping from fighting stance.

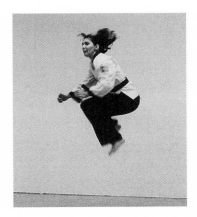

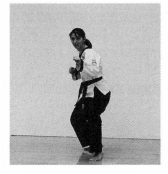

Upper Body Power

Most women have much stronger lower bodies than they have upper bodies. Having strong legs is definitely an advantage in the martial arts, but it is also important to develop upper body strength. Many martial arts, such as Aikido and judo, rely heavily on upper body strength. Karate and Tae Kwon Do performance can be enhanced with improved upper body strength as well. Having confidence in your hand techniques, which is where upper body strength is crucial, can help with your sparring and self-defense practice.

Using Your Entire Body

The most common mistake martial artists make when using hand techniques is to use only their arms to generate power. Often a punch is thrown forward from the shoulder. The only power behind such a punch is the power of your arm. If you lack upper body strength, your punches will therefore be weak and ineffective. An immediate improvement can be made by putting the power of your whole body behind a hand technique. This means using your hips as a pivot point instead of relying only on your shoulder.

Try chambering your fist near your waist. As you punch forward, twist the same side hip forward as well. You should notice a difference right away. Stepping into the punch is another way of putting body power behind a hand technique. You can practice stepping or sliding into a punch as well as turning or pivoting your hip into it. If you combine both hip turning and stepping into the punch, you can create very powerful strikes immediately, without having to increase your muscle mass.

A good way to measure your performance is to punch a heavy bag. Use bag gloves or sparring equipment to protect your hands at first if you haven't been doing much bag work. Try punching the bag just using your arm from the shoulder down. Then try twisting your hips into the punch. Next, step or slide forward as you punch. You should notice a difference in power. To gain the most from these aids, practice punching the heavy bag at least a few minutes each day. Also try different hand techniques as well—knife hands, ridge hands, backfists and the like. These will require slight modifications to your footwork. If no heavy bag is available, use a makiwara board (striking post). Many martial arts schools have these in the training hall. While they aren't as forgiving as heavy bags, they do help condition your hands so that punching and other hand techniques will cause fewer injuries to your hands.

With a little practice, using your whole body to power your punches can make a dramatic difference in your skill.

Boxing

Punching the heavy bag will certainly increase strength in your upper body. If you're interested, adding some boxing drills and skills can make your heavy bag workout more interesting and more productive. While jabs, crosses, hooks and uppercuts aren't always taught at martial arts schools, they are useful technique to know (and not least because you might run across one of them outside the training hall!) Understanding and practicing the techniques of boxing will improve your upper body strength and will help you increase the power of your hand techniques. Many communities have boxing clubs or classes that can teach you the fundamentals. If these are not available, try consulting boxing instruction guides, which can show you basic boxing techniques. Videos are also a good source of information. Finally, many martial arts schools have one or two students who have studied boxing and would be happy to show you some of the basics.

Improving Upper Body Strength

Sometimes the old-fashioned methods of building strong bodies work best. Nothing quite compares to pushups for strengthening your upper arms and chest muscles. Don't be embarrassed to start at the very beginning with these. With your knees on the floor and palms flat, try ten or fifteen pushups twice a day. As you get better, lift your knees off the floor, resting only your toes and palms on the floor. Once you've mastered this, move onto the old martial arts standby—the knuckle pushup. Instead of placing palms down on the floor, make your hands into fists and rest your weight on your first two knuckles (your punching knuckles). This technique will dramatically increase your wrist strength. This helps keep your wrists from rolling when your strike with your hands. Wrists that roll or twist can sprain quite easily. Once you are doing 10 or 15 knuckle pushups comfortably, you have increased your upper body strength considerably. Add to the number of repetitions in increments of five.

If a chin-up (also called pull-up) bar is available, practice these as well. Women are often embarassed to find that they can't even do one chin up and so don't even try. Since these are a great way to improve upper body strength, don't give up. Have a partner act as a spotter at first, helping you to perform your chin-ups. Try for two or three at first, relying less and less on your partner's help each time. Once you can do five without a spotter's help, you have improved your upper body condition considerably. Try increasing the number of chin-ups you do in increments of two or three. Be careful to do this technique correctly; it puts a great deal of strain on your shoulders.

Also, take every opportunity to lift and carry things, from bags of groceries to suitcases to children. Think about upper body strength in your daily life as well as at the training hall. Reach, lift, carry, and move with your upper body (always remember to lift correctly, using your knees, so that you do not strain your back).

Weight Training

Lifting weights is a sure way to improve your upper body strength. The main drawback is that we usually think you have to belong to a fitness club or invest in an expensive home weight machine to lift weights. Not true! Weights for use at home can be very inexpensive. I'm not referring to the weights your strap onto your wrists and do housework in (that's a dangerous practice), nor am I referring to the old women's magazine advice of lifting soup cans to improve your biceps (please). I'm referring to a simple pair of dumbbells, which, with up to fifty or sixty pounds of weight each can be purchased for less than fifty dollars. I have seen 110-pound weight sets for thirty dollars at several sporting goods stores. Make certain that any weight set you purchase is safe to use. Dumbbells are essentially short metal bars upon which plates of various weights are attached. A collar keeps the weights from sliding or moving around as your lift. Be certain that you get a weight set with locking collars for safety. Inspect the bars and the plates. They should be smooth with no burrs or sharp edges. Some people prefer plastic weight plates to metal ones; make certain plastic weight plates are evenly balanced and have no defects.

Simple bicep curls and tricep extensions will do wonders for your upper body. Most weights sets come with instructions for use; remember always to start at a light weight and work your way up. Overdoing weight training or incorrectly practicing can lead to injuries—some very painful and difficult to heal. Therefore, invest in a video or other instruction guide to show you proper technique. Also, some television fitness programs show the proper use of free weights (the name for dumbbells and the like—weights that aren't attached to a machine). You'll also find that a pair of dumbbells can improve your lower body strength; you can use them while performing squats, for instance.

Keep track of your progress in a notebook, recording the amount of weight you are lifting and the number of repetitions. This helps you make steady improvement. If you want to increase your muscle strength without increasing your muscle mass excessively, limit the amount of weight you lift and increase the number of repetitions you perform.

Hand Techniques

Finally, to improve your upper body strength and skills, remember to work with confidence. If you are sparring and you perform a punch, go ahead and punch. Don't just punch tentatively, only to see your technique brushed aside. Striking with confidence is the surest way to improve your upper body techniques.

Using Your Advantages

Although women sometimes find upper body techniques and jumping techniques to be frustrating, all techniques can be mastered with time and practice. There are certain characteristics, however, that put women at a definite advantage in the training hall. These include superior flexibility, speed, agility and kicking. Using these attributes to your advantage can improve your martial arts performance significantly.

Flexibility

Women tend to naturally have more flexibility than men. This is probably because we have, overall, less muscle mass than men. The phrase "muscle-bound" means just that—generally, the bigger the muscles, the less flexibility you have. Of course, some extremely muscular people who pay particular attention to flexibility training can and will retain flexibility, but for the most part, an increase in muscle mass means a decrease in flexibility. This is good to remember, for as you put on muscle mass, perhaps through weight training, aerobic workouts, or martial arts practice, you may find your flexibility decreasing. Therefore, even if you are naturally flexible, keep some stretching and flexibility routines in your workouts.

Because women are naturally more flexible than men on the whole, they enjoy distinct advantages in most martial arts. Also, fitness studies suggest that women *gain* flexibility much more quickly than men, which is related to hormone differences. Your stretches and flexibility training will pay off much sooner than a man's. This certainly helps you stay focused and determined, because improvement is quicker. In addition, these studies suggest that women are able to attain more flexibility overall than their male counterparts can, even if the both men and women begin at the same place. This means men are simply more limited in their flexibility.

Using Flexibility in Martial Arts

For female martial artists, flexibility can be used to overcome disadvantages. For instance, perhaps most of your male sparring partners are taller than you. This means they have longer legs and can reach further than you. But you can neutralize this advantage with your flexibility. You can kick higher than your male partners, for instance. Also, flexibility means you have a greater range of techniques at your disposal. For instance, a crescent or ax kick requires a certain amount of flexibility in the hip and hamstring area. Many men don't have the flexibility required to make this a shoulder or head high kick. But most women do have or can gain this flexibility. Use this range to your advantage. Instead of simply relying on just one or two techniques, develop seven or eight.   Flexibility is also essential in martial arts such as jujutsu, judo and Aikido. Flexibility allows for easier grappling; it also makes you harder to pin. The more flexible you are, the less effective joint locks and the like are on you, and the more easily they are countered. The more flexible you are, the easier it is for you to manipulate others.

Speed

The most important equation for a martial artist to remember is this: mass times speed equals power. This means that a bigger person isn't necessarily more powerful than a smaller person. It means the person who has both mass and speed is more powerful. For this reason, women who are small can still be as powerful as big men; they just have to use speed to their advantage. Again, because women tend to be lighter and less muscular than men, they are in general naturally quicker than men. This speed can translate into power.

Speed Techniques

For this reason, women can use speed techniques in favor of "mass" or muscle techniques to generate power. For instance, a spinning heel kick is a speed technique. It requires speed alone to be effective. If you don't move fast enough, the technique won't work, regardless of how much muscle you have behind it. A reverse side kick, on the other hand, is a mass or muscle technique. Even if you are slow as molasses doing a reverse sidekick, if you have a big body, the technique can be very powerful. Of course, a speed technique, such as the spinning heel kick, can benefit from added strength, just as a muscle technique, such as the reverse sidekick, can be improved with the addition of speed. The two together—mass and speed—are unbeatable.

Speed techniques are excellent for women to use. A spinning backfist can be an excellent hand technique for a woman, as can the whip-like roundhouse kick (which also capitalizes on her flexibility).

Maintaining a Balance

But there is a critical mass. By this, I mean that after a certain amount of muscle or weight is available, the amount of speed also available declines. At a certain weight, speed inevitably declines. This is why you see heavyweight fighters who weigh perhaps two hundred and fifty pounds, but you never see heavyweight fighters who are three hundred and fifty pounds; they are simply too slow and their additional mass cannot overcome this drawback. The great news is that women rarely reach this critical mass, though men reach it much more frequently. Therefore, a woman can lift weights, put on muscle mass and the like as much as she wants without impairing her speed, as long as she keeps practicing for speed.

Acquiring Speed

Speed can be achieved through relaxation—which seems impossible. But consider: the tighter and more clenched your muscles, the slower your techniques will be. Therefore, trying to relax your muscles as you practice your techniques will increase your speed. One way to learn to do this is to try to tighten your muscles as much as possible and then try to relax them as much as possible. Repeat this process several time. This clench-and-release exercise helps you learn what a relaxed muscle feels like. With practice, you'll be able to do controlled, focused, powerful techniques with relaxed muscles and relaxed movements. The more relaxed your muscles are, the faster they move to the target.

At the moment of impact, the muscles should be tightened and the movement should be forceful. This leads to quick and powerful techniques. In addition, adding a whip or snap movement to the end of each technique will increase speed and power. This is why snapping or whip-like techniques, such as a roundhouse kick or a backfist, can be both quick and powerful. The snap or whip movement is accomplished by the quick return or recoil of the technique. For instance, when you punch and land your punch solidly, you will have a powerful technique. But if you punch, and, after landing your punch, quickly return your hand to the starting position, you'll be creating a snap at the end of your technique. You can practice adding a snap to any of your techniques by focusing on quickly returning your hand or foot to its starting or chamber position as soon as your strike has landed.

Maintaining Speed and Quickness

The great enemy of speed is fat, so the less you have, the faster you are. Speed is one of those traits that depend a great deal on your physical condition. If you feel bloated, ate too much for lunch, have the flu—

you'll definitely have less speed than usual. But these ill effects can be countered somewhat by the continual practice of speed techniques. Then, your off days won't be quite so disastrous. But do remember that eating right, sleeping well, and drinking enough water to keep hydrated are all essential to health, fitness—and speed.

By practicing these approaches, you can immediately increase your speed. Over time, these exercises and approaches can significantly improve your quickness.

Agility

Another quality female martial artists can take advantage of is greater agility, which, in a way, is simply a combination of speed and flexibility. Taking advantage of greater agility can improve your martial arts practice, especially in the area of sparring. An agile fighter can avoid getting hit through body movements and footwork. An agile fighter can also defend better, by blocking and countering quickly and accurately. In other areas, agility is important as well. The more advanced martial arts techniques require greater agility. High kicks, flashy or exciting techniques, and complicated movements can be mastered by those practitioners who possess above average agility. Also, the performance of forms requires agility; in more advanced kata or hyung, agility is necessarily if you don't want to lose your balance and fall over.

Using Agility

To capitalize on your natural (or acquired) agility, practice is needed. Repetition improves your agility, but also shows you how to use it to your advantage. In sparring, the main areas to practice are body movement (or body shifting) and footwork. The more agile you are, the easier it is to use body movement and footwork to your advantage.

Body Movement/Body Shifting

Body movement, also called body shifting, is simply a matter of turning your upper body or pivoting on one foot to avoid a strike. Accomplished sparrers can twist at the waist to let a punch or kick slide by and can then follow up with a countering technique of their own. To practice this, instead of blocking your opponent's techniques, try simply shifting your body out of the way (without taking steps). Don't make big, overcommitted movements. The more subtle your body movements, the more effective they will be.

Footwork

In addition, footwork can help your sparring as well. By stepping away from a punch or kick, you can often avoid being struck while at the same time setting up the perfect target for your own technique. Footwork varies according to your martial arts discipline, but three simple patterns are common: stepping left, stepping right and triangular stepping. The first two are self-explanatory; the trick is knowing which direction to step so that you are stepping away from your opponent's technique instead of stepping into it. This footwork can be practiced in much the same way as body movement. Instead of physically blocking the opponent's techniques, simply step away from them. As you grow more comfortable, add your own strikes or techniques after you've stepped out of the way.

Triangular stepping is also what it sounds like—learning to step in a triangle, as opposed to the more common linear method. This means stepping back, to the side, then in or stepping to the side, to the back and then in. Again, each variation requires practice; the more quickly you can move, the better off you'll be. Triangle stepping is an excellent technique to use against opponents who anticipate stepping left or right. It is also helps you avoid your opponent's techniques while putting you inside quickly, where you can land your own techniques.

Agility and Martial Arts Practice

Agility is also useful outside the sparring ring, particularly in the performance of forms. Here, repeated practice of your form will allow your agility to shine through, because agility is linked, in part, to self-confidence.

Use your agility to improve your techniques overall. The best way to do this is through slow motion movements. Again, it seems contrary to say agility comes through slow practice, but slow motion practice actually tunes fine motor muscles and also significantly improves your balance, which is essential to all martial arts. Practice each of the fundamental or basic kicks, moving as slowly as possible from start to finish. Some people count to ten or twenty as they move from beginning to end. Your goal is to execute a technique—a kick or punch—as slowly as possible while still maintaining excellent balance and a smooth, polished technique. This can be very difficult to do, but it is certainly rewarding. It improves agility and it also increases muscle strength and improves balance.

Kicks

Slow motion practice of kicks is good for your agility—and it's also good for perfecting your kicks. By performing slow motion kicks in front of a mirror, you can practice kicking the perfect kick. You can make sure your technique is correct, making adjustments as needed, and you can check to be sure your body line is appropriate and that your kick is as accurate as possible.

Kicking techniques are also among women's strengths. Most women tend to have very powerful lower bodies, especially as compared to upper bodies. Therefore, women can often capitalize on this quality and take advantage of kicking techniques to improve their martial arts practice.

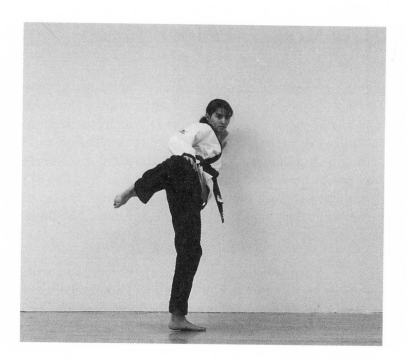

Kicking Variety

One of the most productive things a female martial artist can do is to develop a strong repertoire of kicks. Many martial artists rely on just a few kicks, especially in sparring, but this can be a weakness. The roundhouse kick, side kick and reverse sidekick seem to be the favorite. Since women have speed, flexibility and agility, they should be able to become comfortable enough with almost any kick to add it to their sparring arsenal. Therefore, be sure to add a front kick, crescent or ax kick, reverse crescent kick, and hooking kick to your sparring. Also, think in terms of double kicks; that is, try doing a roundhouse kick to the middle section, then immediately do a roundhouse kick to the high section without setting your leg down. This draws your opponent's guard down, allowing you to score with your roundhouse kick to the high section.

Speed, flexibility and agility will all enhance your kicking ability, so taking advantage of these natural skills will greatly improve your martial arts practice.

Improving Martial Arts Techniques

For optimum performance, you need to build speed, power and endurance. There's nothing mysterious about how this is done—it simply requires a lot of hard work. Speed is acquired through practice and through plyometric drills that help you develop explosive quickness. Power is developed through weight-training and isometric exercises (crunches, push ups). Endurance is developed through the continual practice of pushing yourself even when you are tired. Running and other aerobic exercises can help you build endurance. Chapter Seven describes these fitness elements in more detail.

As you work to gain speed, power, and endurance, you will need to continue perfecting your martial arts techniques. Sometimes as we move up through the ranks we discontinue working on fundamental techniques and focus only on mastering the intermediate or advanced techniques that we are learning. Or we quit trying to master a technique that continually gives us trouble. While no one can perform every martial art technique they are taught flawlessly and perfectly, to give up on techniques because they seem impossible is not the best attitude to take. Sometimes it is just a matter of trying another approach or practicing a little bit differently. Sometimes when we are frustrated, we close ourselves off to the coaching that could help us to succeed, or we quit practicing just when we were about to master the technique. For me, this happened when I was learning various punching combinations that I practiced faithfully on the heavy bag. I could jab and cross but I couldn't add an uppercut that was powerful and effective no matter what my coach said. So I quit trying. I began focusing on different aspects of my martial arts training, and didn't work on my boxing skills for months. Then, a few months after I was awarded my first dan, I went back to the heavy bag to practice some boxing skills, and my uppercut followed my cross perfectly, as if I had been doing it all my life. All I can say is that I was very close to mastering the technique when I gave up on it. I wonder how much better I would be if I hadn't stopped practicing the technique for almost two years.

When I became pregnant, I learned another lesson. I had to modify my workouts slightly—no more sparring, no jumping kicks if I might lose my balance and fall, no takedowns. Other advanced techniques were out of the question because they were too dangerous. So I found myself focusing on all the fundamental techniques I had been taught my first year. During target kicking practice, I worked on my front kick, instead of the jumping 360-degree reverse kick that I liked so well. Instead of tornado kicks, I practiced crescent kicks. I practiced lower belt forms repeatedly while other class members were sparring. And I am certain that taking the opportunity to really work on fundamental techniques has improved my skills. Now I take at least one day (or class) each week for work on fundamentals. During this time, I work on the three basic stances, making sure that are wide and deep. I practice the four or five basic kicks carefully, paying special attention to pivoting correctly and chambering properly. This attention to fundamentals has greatly improved all of my intermediate and advanced techniques.

Don't neglect these basic techniques in favor of devoting all of your attention to the flashier, more exciting advanced techniques.

7

Physical Concerns

Many women practice the martial arts for fitness and weight control. A sensible eating plan and regular exercise prevent many diseases, promote good health and make you feel better. (Remember to see your physician before starting a fitness program, including a martial arts program, especially if you have been sedentary in the past.)

In addition to your martial arts training, you may wish to consider weight training. This may help improve your martial arts performance, plus improve and increase muscle and bone mass. Weight lifting won't necessarily cause you to bulk up. Instead, you can lift weights to define your muscles and increase your strength, without having arms as big as your waist. A weight lifter who is attempting to build mass tries to lift the maximum amount of weight possible for perhaps four or five repetitions, until his or her muscles "fail." This tears down and rebuilds the muscle fibers, causing the bulky look associated with weight lifting. But you can achieve many of the benefits of weight lifting without the bulkiness if you reduce the amount of weight you lift and increase the number of repetitions. This leads to a more streamlined, better defined body.

Some martial artists find additional aerobic exercise to be helpful, as well. Brisk walking or jogging will help build the endurance you need to be a better, more successful martial artist. Sometimes, depending on one's school, the martial arts program may or may not be very aerobic, so it pays to supplement the martial arts workout with an aerobic workout. One way you can determine if your martial arts class is aerobic is to observe what goes on. Does the class permit much observation, correction, and so forth? You're probably cooling down, not keeping your heart rate up. Is the exercise so vigorous that you have to pause to catch your breath? That's anaerobic. But that doesn't mean your martial arts practice has no aerobic benefit. Many martial arts classes can be aerobic if the participant tries to maintain an aerobic heart rate for at least twenty minutes, and still be able to talk while participating in the class.

Your target aerobic heart rate is identified by subtracting your age from 220, and multiplying the result by 50 to 80% depending on how fit you currently are. About 70% is appropriate for most healthy people. Therefore, if you are thirty years old and in good shape, you would multiply 190 (220-30) by .70 (70% of your maximum heart rate) to come up with 133, which is your target heart rate. Your goal, then, would be to work up to that heart rate and continue to work out, keeping your heart rate at about 133 for at least 20 minutes. An easy way to check your pulse rate is to press your fingers against either side of your neck (not too hard—you don't want to cut off the blood flow!) Also, heart rate monitors can be purchased at sporting goods stores. Some of these fit on the tip of your finger, while others can be worn like a watch. These can be used to determine your heart rate without having to stop your workout. By combining some weight training and aerobic exercise with your martial arts practice, you'll be well on your way to optimum health and fitness.

But remember to start training gradually and to add weight and aerobic elements to your workout schedule slowly, over a period of time. Go ahead and attend class once or twice a week, building up to three or four times each week. Don't overdo the intensity of your training. Most martial artists agree that working out every day is what keeps them at their peak. However, always allow a day or two off each week to give your body a break and to let it recuperate from the small tears, aches, pains, and strains that accumulate over time. Participating in a formal martial arts class for an hour or so three times a week will keep you sharp and in shape especially if you supplement that with practice at home. Remember to be realistic.

You may find your body can do more than you ever imagined, but try not to get frustrated if your body doesn't respond as quickly as you would like.

Many women who begin training in the martial arts have little athletic experience. Because the martial arts seem to offer more than just a workout, women who don't consider themselves athletes often join a school. Martial arts isn't just about physical fitness, so sometimes we overlook the amount of stress martial arts can put on our bodies, and especially in the case of non-athletes, it's easy to get injured without realizing that most martial arts injuries can be prevented. Starting slowly and building up to a level of exercise that keeps you fit is the best way to prevent beginner injuries.

Injury Prevention

Although most martial artists talk about injuries as if they are inevitable, being sensible can prevent some of the most common injuries. Warming up, stretching, and cooling down are essential to avoiding injuries. Also, keep in mind that women are more prone to certain injuries than men are. This means it's important to follow stretching techniques for women, not just for men.

Women tend to have a different weight distribution from men. This means that certain injuries are more common to women than to men. Hip injuries are far more frequent among women than men while men have more trouble with hamstring and groin pulls. Also, because women have much stronger legs than arms, it pays to use your legs. However, this emphasis on leg techniques can lead to leg injuries. Overall, the most common injuries in martial arts practice are overuse injuries, hyperextension injuries, and sprains and strains.

Overuse Injuries

Overuse injuries, especially for beginners or for those who are training hard for competition or for rank testing, can be debilitating. Overuse injuries occur when a joint is used repetitively, especially if the joint has not been used extensively before. Overuse injuries like tendinitis and bursitis can cause pain and discomfort in a joint such as a hip, when an individual begins rotating the hip more than usual. To prevent this, be certain to stretch before training. Also, be certain to execute techniques precisely. On a turning kick, if you don't pivot correctly, you'll put undue stress on your hips and knees, which can cause strains, overuse injuries, and ligament damage.

Overuse injuries can be painful and result in frustration, but they rarely cause more than temporary discomfort. If you suspect you have an overuse injury, check with your physician. Visiting with a sports medicine specialist or even a sports trainer can help you to learn how to prevent such problems.

Usually rest, ice, and an anti-inflammatory such as ibuprofen (or in more extreme cases, a prescription medication) will take care of the problem. If not, an injection of cortisone and/or a course of physical therapy may be recommended. Cortisone injections are not painful or scary if you simply relax while the shot is being administered, but it's better for your body if you prevent injuries rather than treat them.

While all joints can be affected, for women hips and knees are most commonly overused, followed by shoulder overuse injuries. Why shoulders? Well, because most women don't have the same amount of upper body strength as their male counterparts. Since martial arts advocate a variety of hand, elbow and arm techniques, one's shoulders are stressed and strained differently than usual. Since the muscle mass is usually not as well-developed here as in other parts of the body, these stresses and strains are more likely to cause an injury, especially an overuse injury. Overuse injuries include bursitis, tendinitis, plus strains, tears and stress fractures. Remember to stretch all of your joints—including your shoulders—before you start training.

Hyperextension Injuries

Hyperextension occurs when a joint is forced to move beyond its usual stopping point. This can happen when a punch or kick is thrown with full energy but no target exists to absorb the energy of the strike. For instance, kicking the heavy bag will rarely cause a hyperextension injury because the energy and power of the kick is absorbed by the heavy bag. The heavy bag then receives the stress of the kick instead of your ankle, knee or hip joint. But when you kick in the air without using a heavy bag or target, such as when you do repetitive practice in training class or in front of a mirror, your energy isn't absorbed by anything outside your body. To prevent hyperextension, many martial artists recommend that you keep the joint slightly bent—never fully extend a joint for full power unless you are using the heavy bag.

Hyperextension is easily identified. If you suddenly have pain in a joint after you execute a technique, and the pain persists whenever you use the affected limb, you may have hyperextended a joint. Rest, ice, anti-inflammatories—and, if pain continues or worsens—a visit to the doctor are all called for.

Acute Injuries

Sprains, strains and tears, cuts and bruises are all very similar in origin and effect. While overuse injuries have to do with using a joint or limb too much over the course of a certain amount of time—they are cumulative, in effect—strains, sprains, tears, cuts and bruises are all usually the result of an acute injury—that is, a single event that happens suddenly and causes an injury. Perhaps you land wrong on your foot, roll your ankle and end up with a sprain. Or you attempt to improve your flexibility too quickly and suddenly you've got a tear in your hamstring. Sprains and strains can range from mild to severe. The milder cases require little attention, perhaps some aspirin and some ice. More serious cases require rest, ice, compression and elevation, a treatment also known by its acronym "RICE."

1) Strain

A pulled muscle or muscle strain is usually the result of a specific injury, with pain, tenderness and swelling the usual signs. If the muscle doesn't seem to work at all, seek treatment immediately—the muscle itself may have ruptured, in which case, surgery may be necessary to repair it.

A muscle strain happens when a muscle is overstretched or overworked. The muscle continues to function—it just becomes sore. More serious strains may result in muscle tears, which require more time and rest to heal. In martial arts, the most common strains occur in the hamstring and the groin area. For women, the hip flexors are commonly affected. Most strains are quick to mend. The area should be iced on and off for 24 hours, then a heating pad can be used. Some people prefer to ice a strained muscle the entire time it is injured. A few days of rest is usually all that is needed. More serious strains may benefit from an anti-inflammatory or muscle relaxant. For this, consult your physician. To prevent such strains, be certain to warm up and stretch before working out. Also, if you are prone to strains, incorporate weight training and other conditioning exercises into your fitness program.

2) Sprain

A sprain, a word that is often used to identify what is actually a strain or pull, is in fact an injury to the ligaments that connect muscles to bones. Usually a twist, a misstep or an extreme stretch puts too much strain on the ligaments, and tissue is torn. The ankles, knees and even the arches are the most common areas to sustain a strain. Rapid swelling, reduced ability to use the affected area and pain all signal a sprain. If you actually hear a snapping sound, seek treatment immediately, stopping only to apply ice to the area. This snapping sound may indicate a detached ligament, an injury called "window shading." The ligament is torn from the bone and pops away, resulting in a snapping sound. Surgery is sometimes needed to repair the damage.

For routine sprains, ice, compression and rest will cure the condition. The sprained part can usually bear weight after a day or two, but remember this doesn't mean it is completely healed. For a few weeks, minimize your workout intensity to avoid exacerbating the sprain. If the sprain is severe or the joint is unstable, the area may need to be immobilized with a cast or splint.

Physical therapy can help you regain a full range of motion. If you repeatedly sprain a certain joint, use a brace, wrap or tape to help support the area and prevent progressive weakening of and even eventual destruction of the joint. Also, consult your physician, who can recommend a sports trainer or a physical therapist for tips on preventing recurring injuries.

3) Cramps

Muscle cramps, while not exactly an injury, often occur, causing pain and discomfort for the martial artist. Sudden sharp pain or lumps of muscle tissue that can be seen or felt indicate a muscle cramp. These can happen when the muscle is injured or overused. Fatigue and dehydration can contribute to cramps. Usually, muscle cramps are just an inconvenience that will go away without any special treatment. If they occur frequently or interfere with your sleep, consult your doctor. Sometimes a compressed nerve will cause muscle cramps, as will potassium loss, although these are rare conditions.

To treat a cramp, stretch the contracted area. This should provide some relief from the pain. Then massage the muscle, applying pressure. Compression, heating pads and a long soak in a warm bath can help as well. Some people find that ice packs are helpful. To prevent muscle cramps, stretch thoroughly before and after working out, drink plenty of fluids and don't over do it.

4) Cuts and Bruises

Bruises and cuts are probably the most common martial arts related injuries. Usually, some ice or a bandage will suffice. For more serious cases, a visit to the doctor may be needed. Bleeding that won't stop is a sign to seek medical help. Bleeding from the nose, particularly after trauma to the nose should be checked, especially if swelling occurs. A cracked or broken nose can interfere with breathing, and a physician can help it heal correctly. Probably the most common martial arts bruise is the thigh bruise; this can cause pain and swelling, can interfere with bending the knee and cause muscle cramping. Though painful, a thigh bruise will eventually heal on its own. Rest, ice, compression, and elevation can help. It is not unusual to even need crutches to keep the weight off a badly bruised thigh. All for just a bruise! You'll want to see a doctor if the injury doesn't improve or there's the possibility of a fracture. Use pads when sparring to lessen bruising and cuts. When practicing take down moves, as in Aikido, practice on mats that cushion the fall.

5) Fractures

Fractures can be obvious or less obvious; pain, loss of function, swelling and change in the look of a bone all indicate the possibility of a fracture. If you have such symptoms, you should get treatment immediately. When I broke my arm, it took me several days to visit the doctor, because I simply thought I had hyperextended my elbow and the pain, discomfort and difficulty of use would go away. (This is an example of denial that happens to most athletes sooner or later.) Since severe sprains and minor fractures are similar in appearance and pain, x-rays may be taken to determine what has happened. Even x-rays, however, cannot always confirm or contradict a diagnosis, and often severe sprains and minor fractures are treated the same anyway. Some fractures, such as with the small bones of the feet or hands, cannot be treated very effectively, except by resting the affected area. Sometimes the injured finger or toe will be taped to the one next to it, simply to provide additional support and prevent further trauma.

A few weeks may be sufficient for a fracture to heal although it may take a few months. A bone break may need to be set using screws or plates. Usually, the broken bone must be kept immobile, commonly through the use of a cast or splint. Traction and bed rest are used only when a broken bone is difficult to keep immobile, such as a pelvic bone.

A fractured bone often requires physical therapy treatment. Otherwise, muscle tone is lost, stiffness occurs and healing is slower.

6) Stress Fractures

Stress fractures, like other overuse injuries, can occur over time. A bone that must withstand repeated blows may sometimes develop a break or a series of small fissures that have the effect of a fracture. In martial arts these kinds of fractures occasionally occur, usually in a foot or hand. Using proper technique and limiting the amount of abuse you direct toward any one area of your body can help prevent such an injury. A stress fracture can feel similar to a broken bone, or it can feel like a simple overuse injury.

7) Dislocations

Dislocations usually occur after acute injury, that is, a one-time event that directly causes the injury. A dislocation occurs when the ends of the bones of the joint slip out of their normal place and position. This causes pain, swelling and difficulty using the affected joint. Sometimes a dislocation will injure nearby muscles and ligaments. People with certain diseases, such as rheumatoid arthritis, are more inclined to have this happen. Again, seeking treatment immediately is essential to distinguish a dislocation from a fracture, to determine the extent of damage and to prevent further damage to the surrounding tissues. Usually the dislocation is easily corrected and the area is immobilized for a few days. After this, physical therapy can help bring the affected area back to full use.

Do not resume full speed training until your physician has cleared it. You can reinjure the joint, and even cause permanent damage and disability. Physical therapy may also help strengthen the surrounding muscles and ligaments to prevent a recurrence of a dislocation.

8) Back Injuries

Injuries and strains to the back should always be treated with care because of the possible involvement of the spinal column. Spinal cord injuries are actually quite rare in most sports, and are especially rare in the martial arts, but ruptured disks and the like may occur. Any sharp pain in the back should be heeded. Unexplained tenderness or swelling may be signs of concern and should be checked out as well.

Although it is not uncommon to have an injury, they can often be prevented if you use your common sense. Any fitness program should include certain stages—the warm-up, stretching, the exercise itself, and the cool-down. In many martial arts schools, you'll be responsible for your own warming up, stretching and cooling down. If this is the case at your school, try to arrive a few minutes early to prepare for class (check to make sure you are allowed.) Plan to stay a few minutes after to cool down, again if possible. If you can't use the facility this way (for instance, other classes are going on) try to do your warming up and cooling down in the locker room area.

Warming Up

The warm-up period allows your cold muscles a chance to get ready before you put a lot of stress on them. This period will help you obtain, improve and keep your flexibility. Since flexibility is essential to martial arts practice, this time should be used wisely to capitalize on its potential. A good warm-up will help prevent injury, and can also go a long way toward preventing muscle stiffness and soreness. Begin by walking briskly or jogging slowly. As soon as you begin to sweat, you may begin light stretching. Hold each stretch for ten to thirty seconds. No bouncing. If you feel pain, ease up! You should feel the stretch, not pain. Give yourself at least five minutes for stretches—preferably ten. Do stretch all the major muscle groups. Think of going from top to bottom or bottom to top— feet, calves, knees, thighs, hips, back, shoulders, elbows, hands, neck.

If you have arthritis in a joint or have more difficulty using one muscle group over others, spend additional time loosening up that area. If you are nursing an overuse injury, spend additional time warming up that area. If you have a joint or muscle that gives you trouble, try wearing a support—not a wrap. If you put a wrap on too tightly, you can really hurt yourself; plus, the material in ACE-type bandages gets wet when you sweat, and the wraps don't hold up well under lots of action. They unravel and cause distractions. Buy a neoprene support instead. They support your joint or muscle, keep the heat in and don't get soggy when wet. These are available for ankles, knees, elbows, wrists, and hands. Sometimes they are more readily available from business supply catalogs than sporting goods stores because workers often use these supports to prevent injury on the job (while lifting boxes, for instance). Use a lumbar support belt if your back gives your trouble. I have even located and used a pair of neoprene shorts that helped me continue to practice after I developed bursitis in one hip. The compression and support helped keep me from re-injuring the hip and gave the joint additional stability.

Keep your muscles warm by keeping in motion until the start of class. Then you can participate with more intensity, without hurting yourself. During the class, you may do additional stretching exercises. Take advantage of these and improve your flexibility by stretching a little further, a little more completely, than you did during your warm up period. Don't bounce and don't overdo the stretch!

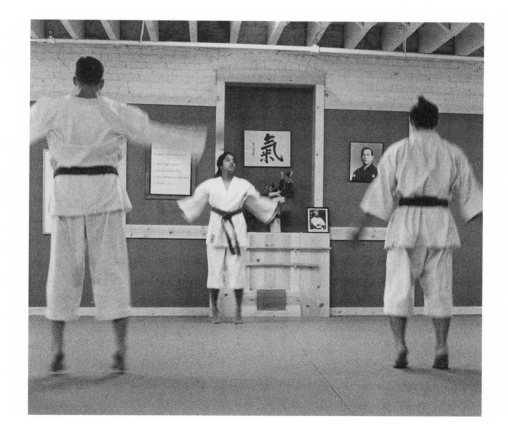

Warming-up and cooling down are essential parts of every workout.

Cooling Down

When class is over, or during breaks that may occur, don't just stop and sit down. Allow for a cool-down period. Your needn't continue aerobic activity, but remember to stretch. Again, to help prevent muscle soreness and stiffness, a cool-down period is highly recommended. Walking or light stretching will help your body return to normal without the undue stress associated with abruptly stopping a workout and coming to a complete rest. Spend five or ten minutes cooling down. Do some of the same stretches you did before the start of class. Some martial artists practice their techniques slowly and gently during the cool down period. This helps them to perfect the techniques they have been working on throughout the class while doing something good for their bodies.

Some stretches that can be used before and after class include those on the following pages. These stretches are just to get you started. You may find others that you prefer, or that work better for your particular needs. But remember, proper stretching is essential. Don't overstretch and don't bounce while stretching. Never continue a stretch if you feel pain. All stretches should be done slowly and precisely. Make attending martial arts classes or working out on your own a priority. The more you remain in an exercise habit, the more your body becomes accustomed to the demands you make on it, and the less likely you are to injure it.

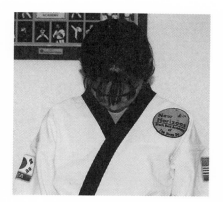
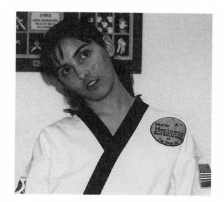
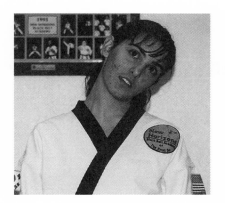
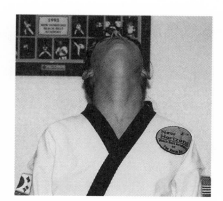

Neck Stretch

Instead of rotating your head in all directions, which can cause pinched nerves, stretch your neck in each of the four directions. Tuck your chin toward your chest, until you feel the stretch. Then hold for ten seconds, relax and repeat. Next, tilt your head to the left, trying to touch your ear to your shoulder. Hold for ten seconds, relax and repeat. Then tilt your head to the right, hold, and repeat. Finally, tilt your head back, so that you are staring at the ceiling, hold for ten seconds, relax and repeat.

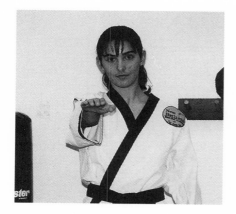 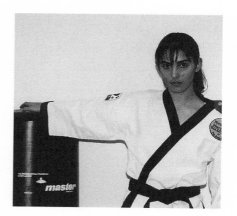

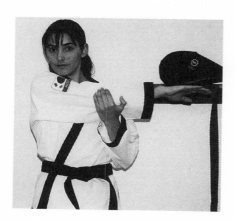 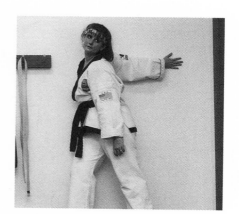

Shoulder Stretch

Extend your arm horizontally to the floor. Bring it across your chest until you feel the stretch in the back of your shoulder/upper arm. Hold for ten seconds, then relax and repeat. Then, arm still horizontal to the ground, reach to the back (without twisting at the waist). Hold for ten seconds, then relax and repeat. Do each stretch three or four times for each shoulder.

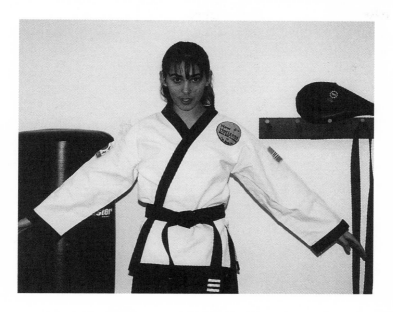

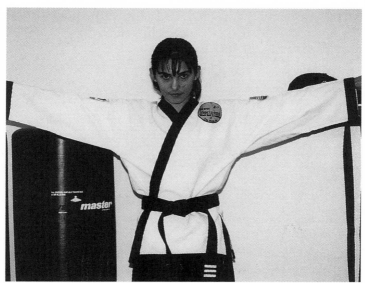

Arm Rotation

With both arms extended horizontally to the ground, make circles with your hands, going forward, then backward. Work slowly, stretching the muscles, not bouncing them or rotating quickly.

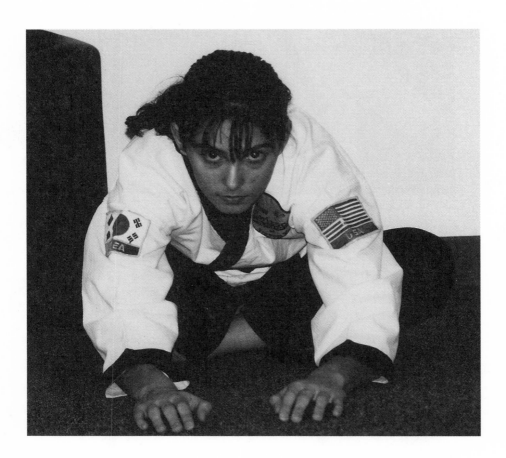

Back Stretches

Sit on the floor with your legs crossed. Keeping your body straight, gently bend toward the floor. The idea is to touch your chin to your legs, but again, don't overstretch. Do as much as feels comfortable. Reach your maximum stretch (no bouncing!). Hold for ten seconds, relax and repeat. To stretch your shoulders at the same time, put your arms in front of you, bend them at the elbows, and hold them together. Then bend, touching your elbows to the floor.

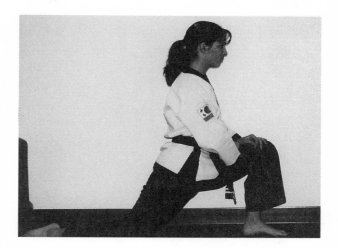

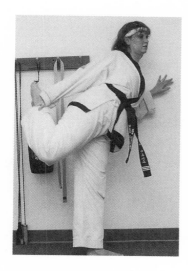

Hip Flexor Stretch

The flexor muscle is on top of the hip, running from the lower abdomen to the thigh. This muscle is easily strained in women, so stretch it thoroughly. Kneel with one knee on the floor. The other knee should be bent at a 90 degree angle, foot flat on the floor. Slowly roll your hip forward so that you feel the stretch on top of your hip and thigh. Support yourself by placing your hands on the floor; putting hands on hips or knees causes too much stress. Hold the forward position for about ten seconds, then relax and repeat. Switch legs and repeat.

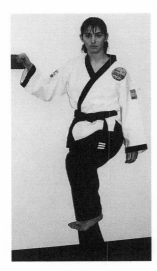

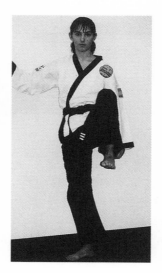

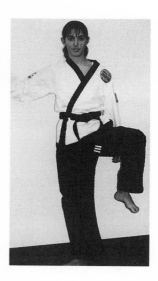

Hip Rotation

Since martial arts practice requires a full range of motion, it is important to work your hips through the full range of motion before working out. Stand near a corner. Brace yourself by planting both palms on opposite walls. Then, lift your leg, bend it at the knee and move it in a full circle. Rotate the leg several times, going slowly and smoothly. Repeat several times on each leg.

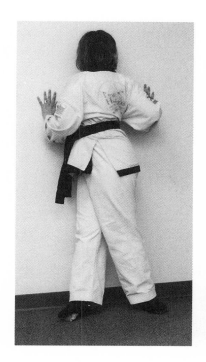

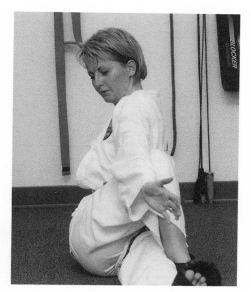

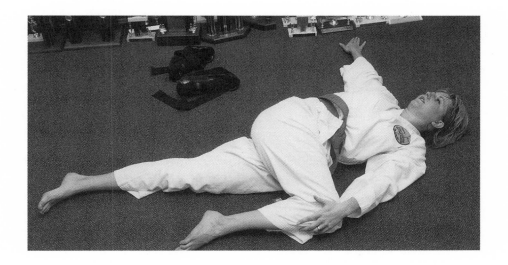

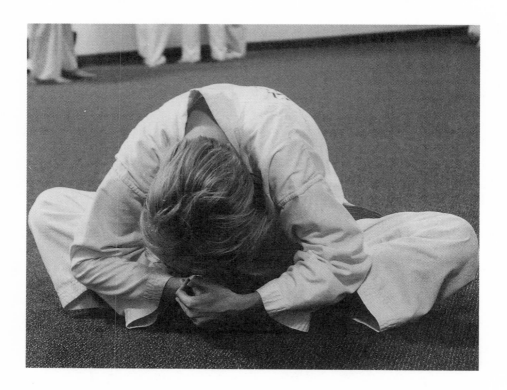

Groin Stretch

Though groin injuries are more common for men than women, you don't want to neglect stretching your groin area. Sit with your legs out in front of you. Slide them toward you until the soles of your feet are touching. Then, continue moving your legs toward you until you feel the stretch. Hold for ten seconds, then relax and repeat. Next, try to touch your knees to the floor by tightening your buttocks muscles (do not use your hands to push your knees or legs). Hold the position as close to the floor as possible for ten seconds, then relax and repeat.

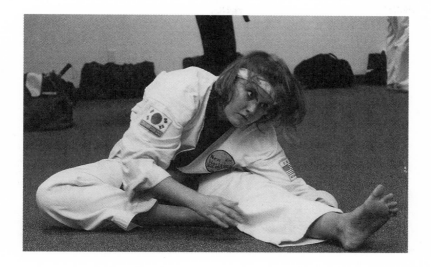

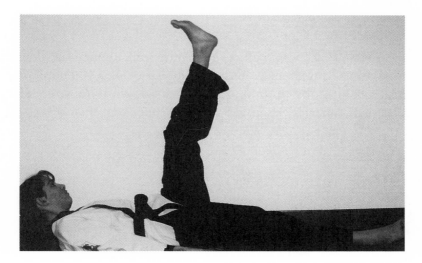

Hamstring Stretch

Lie on your back. Place your hands or a rolled up towel under the small of your back for support. Lift your leg up and extend it at a 90 degree angle to the floor. Then, keeping your leg straight, try to touch your knee to your shoulder. Don't overdo the stretch, and don't bounce. When your leg is at its full stretch, hold for ten seconds, then relax and repeat. Slowly lower your leg to the floor and stretch the other leg.

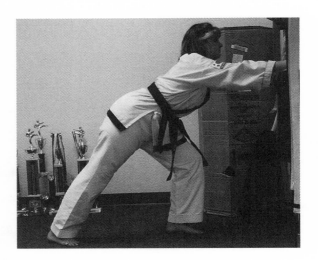

Calf Stretches

Stand facing a wall. Place your palms against the wall, about a shoulder's width apart, elbows bent slightly. Extend your leg behind you until your toes are just touching the ground. Then press down with your heel, stretching the calf muscle. Hold for about ten seconds, then relax and repeat.

Stance Stretches

These stretch several main muscle groups and improve your martial arts techniques at the same time. Position yourself in any of the stances that you have been taught. Then lower your stance until you feel the stretch. Hold for about ten seconds, relax and repeat. Some of the most common stance stretches are the horse stance, the front stance and the back stance. The horse stance is done by placing the feet parallel, about a shoulder's width apart, and bending the knees at a 90 degree angle. The front stance, also known as a forward stance, is done by placing one leg forward, bending the knee at a 90 degree angle, and keeping the back leg straight, with both feet firmly planted on the ground. The back stance is done by keeping both feet on the same line, and bearing most of your weight on the back leg, keeping the heel of the front leg off the floor.

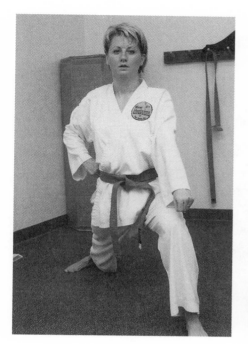

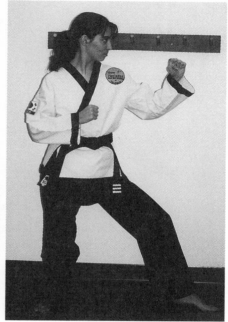

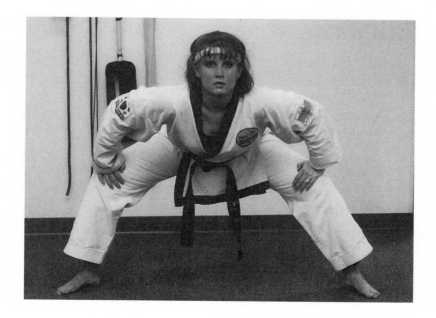

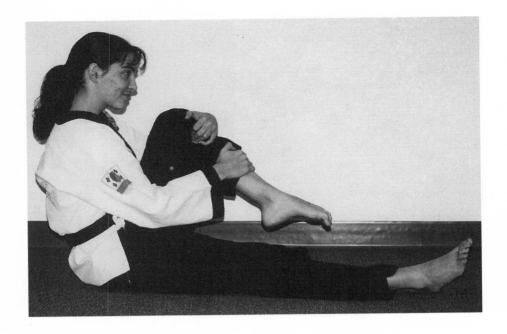

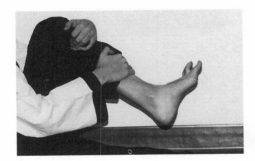 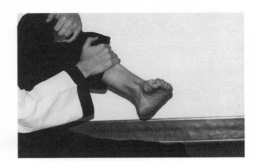

Ankle Rotation

Sitting on the floor, prop your ankle up by crossing your legs. Rotate your ankle in all directions (don't use your hands). Do several rotations with each ankle.

Rehabilitation

If you do get injured, give yourself time to heal. The worst thing you can do is try to come back too soon. Following your doctor's recommendations is essential to full recovery.

Minor injuries always benefit from the RICE treatment, sometimes referred to as the PRICE treatment—protection, rest, ice, compression and elevation. These are the five basic elements that promote healing. Although a nice warm shower or soak in the hot tub will help relieve minor stiffness, warmth encourages swelling, so a soak in the hot tub is exactly what *not* to do in the case of an injury. The only exception to this is when a muscle develops a cramp—then heat will relieve the pain and ease the muscle contraction. After the first twenty-four hours, it is acceptable to use heat to ease pain, stiffness and soreness, but again some people find that using ice throughout the recovery period is preferable, helping them recover more quickly from swelling and tenderness.

Protecting the injured area helps healing and prevents further damage. Bandages, wraps, and slings can be used for this purpose. Canes or crutches can help keep weight off injured legs, ankles and feet.

Rest is essential. Don't do anything that causes pain and/or swelling in the affected area. Most minor injuries will be better after a few days' rest. Not allowing time to rest means the injury never fully recovers and is easily aggravated. Complete healing can take weeks, so don't overdo it.

Ice, of course, decreases pain and swelling. Ice massage and even ice baths can help. Just remember not to allow ice to touch the skin directly—this can cause tissue damage similar to frostbite. Be sure to wrap an ice pack in a clean cloth before applying it to the affected area. An ice bath is actually a slush bath; just as soaking your tired feet at the end of a long day can make you feel better, soaking an injured hand in a slush bath can do wonders to ease pain, swelling and stiffness. Also remember that ice should be applied intermittently. A fifteen minute rest with an ice pack should be followed by forty-five minutes without an ice pack. Then reapply the ice for another fifteen minutes. Especially in the early stage of treatment, mixing ice with no ice helps. Do this often and for at least a few hours after the initial injury. Because swelling reduces your ability to use a joint or limb (not to mention how it hurts) compression is recommended to support the area until swelling subsides. Wraps, such as an ACE bandage, can help. In addition to supporting the swollen area, such wraps can also help protect the injured area.

Finally, elevation is necessary to reduce swelling and prevent tissue damage. Elevate the affected limb so that it is above your heart. This improves blood circulation and also helps reduce swelling. At night, use a pillow or a folded blanket to support and elevate the limb. Protection of the injured limb is also very important at night, when it is easy to reinjure an affected limb by ordinary tossing and turning, or by the ordinary tossing and turning of your partner.

For moderate and severe injures, your doctor may recommend physical therapy sessions. These may be limited to one or two treatments where perhaps you'll be fitted with a splint, or shown how to use an electronic nerve stimulating machine for pain relief (a TENS unit). More often, you might attend several sessions in which your injury is assessed and steps for regaining strength and mobility will be outlined. Special exercises may be shown for you to do at home. Occasionally, ultrasound therapy with a topical anti-inflammatory or pain killer will be used, especially in the case of overuse injuries. Carefully following the therapist's directions will speed you on your way to a quick, complete recovery.

A sports trainer or sports medicine physician has a good understanding of sports injuries and sports rehabilitation. The goal of sports rehabilitation is not only to help you return to normal, but also to help you return to your sports training program. It is essential for martial artists to explain to those who treat them what exactly is involved in their martial arts. Even a physician specializing in sports medicine may have misconceptions about martial arts practice, or may think that all martial arts are like karate, when an art like Aikido or judo is really much different. Inform your health care provider what is actually involved in your training and practice, as this varies widely among the arts. Each art stresses different body parts, different techniques and each requires different degrees of strength and flexibility. For my bursitis, it was important for my therapist to understand how I used my hips (lots of pivots). Upon demonstrating techniques to her, she was able to point out ways I could continue to practice without putting as much stress on my hips. Also, a therapist can give stretching tips.

On another occasion, a physical therapist asked how the injury in my shoulder occurred, and I said I thought it was overuse, from martial arts training. She laughed and did not take the suggestion seriously. (I don't know what she thought martial arts training consisted of). If she had simply asked a question or two, she might have learned that I spend an hour or two after each training sessions punching the heavy bag. It was another martial artist who watched me work out and who helped me understand what I was doing. While boxing against the heavy bag, I was standing too far away from the bag even though I was throwing full force punches each time. I was basically hyperextending my shoulder joint every time I punched. He showed me how to move closer to the bag. This not only improved my punching power, it dramatically improved my shoulder. Three lessons, then:

> 1) Listen to what other martial artists say, especially those you work out with. Ask them how to prevent injuries and how to correct faulty technique.

> 2) You can often continue to train even if you do have an injury. (More on that later.)

> 3) Communicate clearly and effectively with your health care provider.

Falling Correctly

In addition to the common methods for avoiding injury that have been described, consider some other practical steps. If your martial arts style advocates grappling or takedowns, learning to fall will be the best thing you ever do to prevent damage. Certain arts, such as judo, spend much time training practitioners in how to fall, but other styles spend much less time at this and so it is up to you to practice and learn.

Usually, when falling to the back, the tendency is to put your hand out behind you to break your fall. This impulse must be overcome, since it is a good way to injure yourself. Mine is not the only arm that has been broken by falling to the back improperly.

A fall to the back should be absorbed on the hip and the shoulder. Tuck your chin in. Never let the back of your head touch the ground. Practice tucking your head in the mirror; even though you think you are tucking your chin well, you'd be surprised at how you're not. Exaggerate the motion until you have stretched your neck muscles enough to know what a fully, firmly tucked chin feels like. Slap your hand, palm down, on the ground, straightening your arm as you do so. This will help you overcome the tendency to put your hand or arm straight back to break the fall. Bend your arm at the elbow, fall on your shoulder and hip and slap the ground simultaneously. When falling to the front, it is important not to land directly on your hand. Keep your head lifted and use your hand and arm to slide yourself forward. Learn other falling techniques as necessary to prevent injury. Breakfalls, as these are called, vary widely from one style to another.

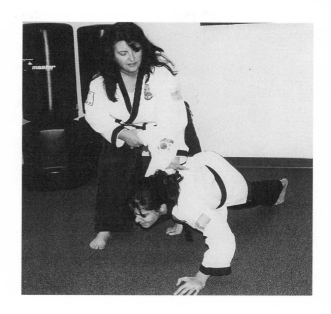

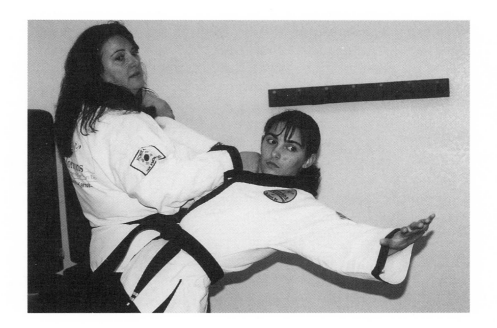

Always support your partner during throwing techniques.

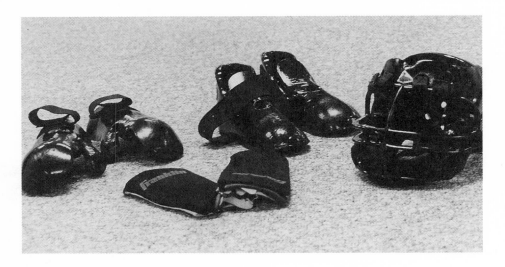

Safety Gear

To prevent injury, wear protective pads, such as sparring gear, if you belong to a style that spars. Although the bare knuckles approach might be increasingly popular in martial arts and is always popular in real fights, you shouldn't practice bare-knuckled except when noncontact sparring, or when working on a sparring technique under carefully controlled conditions. Also, insist that your sparring partners wear sparring equipment (pads). When our school first started using headgear, those of us who were black belts complained bitterly (black belts are always complaining bitterly about something). You couldn't see out of the darned things. We were certain people kicked us harder than before and we even thought headgear made it easier for us to get lazy about protecting our heads. When you get your un-headgeared bell rung once or twice, you learn to keep your hands up. However, the number of broken noses and chipped teeth dropped dramatically after we all started using headgear, so now we are glad to have it. Now we occasionally spar without headgear, but only with partners who have good control or when we are practicing no contact or light contact sparring.

Consider using a heavy bag or striking post if you want to practice without pads, but remember it's easy to roll a wrist when punching, so wrist wraps or bag gloves will help you strengthen your wrists until you develop stronger wrists and hands. Hands and wrists can also be strengthened by doing pushups on your knuckles.

Never wear jewelry in class—no earrings, necklaces, diamond wedding rings, watches or navel rings. These can cause injury to yourself and to others, and they can catch on uniforms and tear them. If your partner is wearing jewelry, it is well within your rights to ask him or her to remove it for your safety.

First Aid

Further, to prevent an injury from becoming a disability or worse, it is important for some members of the martial arts class to be aware of proper first aid procedures. Anyone who leads a class should have at least basic knowledge of first aid. At many schools, everyone who teaches is certified in CPR. It is a good idea for all martial artists to learn CPR and standard first aid. It is the responsible thing to do and it may encourage others who practice with you to become certified. You might suggest to your instructor that a training session be sponsored at your school so that interested martial artists can have a chance to learn. Hospitals, the Red Cross and other health care agencies in your area often offer these classes for little or no cost.

The school should have first aid supplies available, and students should know where the kit is located. Essentials include bandages, disposable rubber gloves, smelling salts, medical scissors, gauze, tape, ACE-type wraps, a first aid manual, and chemical ice packs (which can be stored at room temperature and are activated when a chemical agent inside the bag is released, usually by twisting the bag). Iodine, rubbing alcohol, and aspirin can also be helpful. A blood spill kit, used to clean blood off of equipment, mats or gear, is also becoming a common part of a well-stocked first aid kit. If your school doesn't have a basic first aid kit, consider making one a gift to your instructors.

Pregnancy

Another common concern of female martial artists is what happens when they become pregnant. Can they continue their martial arts practice—and if so, how? Well, the good news is that pregnant women who have exercised regularly before pregnancy can continue to do so during and after pregnancy, though you must remember to keep your workouts reasonable. Exercise will have little impact on your child, though you will reap the rewards of easier labor, faster recovery, and more stamina after delivery.

Remember, however, that pregnancy is not the right time to <u>start</u> a martial arts class or an intense fitness program, if you haven't already been doing so. Also, even if you have been exercising regularly, check with your doctor before continuing to work out at your usual pace.

As your pregnancy progresses, you'll find you'll have to modify what you can do. While certain enviable persons can still kick head high during pregnancy, do not get discouraged if you can't. Above all, don't quit! Just slow down a bit. Once the baby is born, you'll be back to your former level before long. You may even find that your skills have improved.

Again, check with your physician before starting or continuing a fitness program if you become pregnant. Also remember that because of changes in your body, you are more easily injured during pregnancy than at any other time. Your weight distribution and center of gravity shift, making you more likely to lose your balance and fall. More pressure and stress is being put on your joints, so avoid too much weight bearing exercise, and restrict the amount of stress you put on a single joint. Avoid abrupt changes in direction (which can causes falls and other injuries), and don't do high impact workouts. Also, avoid exercises that require you to lie on your back (this could restrict blood flow or oxygen to you or the fetus). It is still important to warm up, stretch and cool down. You may become tired faster—listen to your body. Now is not the time to push it. Also, drink plenty of fluids and avoid working out when it is extremely hot and humid. Discuss your condition with your instructor, including any limitations imposed by your physician.

You will probably want to discontinue sparring as soon as you discover you are pregnant, in order to prevent any accidental blows to your abdomen. Although your baby is well protected by your body, it is best not to risk it. You should also avoid throws and takedowns. This may put a big crimp in a judo practitioner's practice, but remember you can modify everything. Your partner can practice entering and breaking your balance without actually throwing you to the mat—and you can do the same with your partner. Your martial arts practice can be modified in whatever way is necessary. For instance, even if you have to avoid jumping kicks, you can still focus on the fundamentals—front kicks, side kicks, roundhouse kicks—which will help you remain sharp and focused.

Physical Limitations

Although pregnancy is temporary and you'll return to your pre-pregnancy self soon enough, sometimes we develop disorders, diseases or problems that permanently affect our ability to do martial arts. But martial arts can still be practiced. Even if you are disabled, there is no reason you can't take advantage of all that the martial arts have to offer. Most schools are delighted to accommodate disabled individuals, who are also invited to participate in regular martial arts tournament competitions. The physical limitations of the disabled person should be discussed with the main instructor, who can make modifications to the workout and otherwise serve as an advisor for the disabled student and those who work with him or her. Consulting your physician before you begin is also advisable.

Older women and younger girls can also participate without trouble—as usual, check with your physician, especially if you have not been participating in a fitness program recently. Older people may need to undergo an exercise stress test to make certain there are no otherwise undetected heart problems. Girls as young as four and five and women in their seventies and beyond have enjoyed the benefits of martial arts, including cardiovascular fitness, self-confidence and reduced risk of osteoporosis. If chest pain, joint pain or other symptoms appear, discontinue working out and see your physician. Then get his or her permission to return to your fitness program. Most instructors will be accommodating. For instance, in some styles of Tae Kwon Do, board-breaking is a requirement for earning higher belt ranks. But in the case of individuals with certain kinds of disabilities, pads will be substituted so that the individual can demonstrate power and technique without putting excess strain on their bodies.

People with high blood pressure, arthritis and other medical difficulties have all benefitted from participating in martial arts. Make sure your physician understands that you are a martial artist who wishes to continue training. Make certain he or she has a clear understanding of how you train, and what is involved in a typical class. I was told that my hip needed to be replaced and that I had to quit Tae Kwon Do. I was far too young to think about hip replacement surgery, and I didn't want to quit Tae Kwon Do. Finally, I found a physician who understood that I intended to keep working out, and that the benefits of martial arts practice for me far outweighed any of the negatives of making my bursitis worse. This is not to say that you should find a physician who'll just go along with anything you say, or who prescribes medication when in fact changing your fitness program is a better choice. What is important is finding a physician who understands the purpose and the practice of the martial arts.

Even if you are very big or very little, you shouldn't refrain from practicing a martial art. Your physician may suggest modifications to the program, but people of all shapes, sizes and fitness levels have had great success in the martial arts.

On occasion, you may have surgery or some other type of medical condition that will change your ability to practice the martial arts, either temporarily or permanently. Perhaps a chronic disease has been identified, such as asthma, that will affect martial arts performance. Perhaps you are attempting to return to the training hall after the birth or a child, or perhaps a C-section has been performed, and you aren't quite up to speed, or perhaps you had your appendix out or a cyst on your ovary removed—all of these things affect your martial arts training and your martial arts performance. Since women have to cope with pregnancy, ovarian cysts, and the like in addition to the usual health problems, it is likely that an otherwise healthy women will have more medical concerns than an otherwise healthy man. This can be frustrating. You can miss class, miss training and then return only to discover that you have lost all of your flexibility. Some things to keep in mind: always return to physical activity under the advice of a medical doctor. Also, be certain to communicate clearly to your physician what you want to do. Misunderstandings may mean you are prevented from doing things you actually can do with no harm, or that you return to practicing before you should.

Although childbirth and surgery are exhausting experiences, try to think about your martial arts practice even when you are not attending training sessions regularly. You might be able to work in stretches while your ten-year old feeds the new baby under your supervision. You might be able to incorporate weight training into your day by lifting and carrying. You might walk instead of parking the car near the front door of the grocery store.

You might find ways to incorporate the baby and any other children into workouts that are light, short and fun (this is good for the kids too). Or perhaps train a bit with your partner while at home—explain what you want to accomplish and challenge him or her to help get you there.

After surgery, as you feel more and more energetic, add activities that can help you keep your flexibility, speed and strength. Take time to do upper body stretches, for instance, if you've had knee surgery. Stretching, especially light easy stretching, can always be done on areas that are not affected by surgery or injury. Often, while showering or bathing, you can stretch the unaffected muscles and joints to help remain flexible. Aquatic practice is also an excellent way to keep in shape while you recover. Since the buoyancy of the water offers support to injured body parts, you can often work on aerobic and stretching exercises on nearly your entire body while keeping your injured area relatively protected.

Resistance exercises can often be done. You can maintain upper body strength, for instance, without injury to that knee, by acquiring a rubber or elastic band from a medical supply shop or a physical therapist (these often go by the name Theraband). These bands are specifically designed to work as resistance devices; don't substitute something else, such as a homemade device. This could rip, tear or snap back, causing another injury. If it's your arm that's affected, use the band to maintain strength in your legs. If your leg is affected, use the band to maintain strength and flexibility in your arms. You can pull the band in opposite directions to work on upper body strength.

Most martial arts teach forms—series of techniques put together in a prearranged pattern, also called kata or hyung. Slow, careful practice of these forms can help you feel you're maintaining your techniques. If you just had surgery on your knee, don't do deep stances or snap kicks high. Walk through the form, omitting kicks and keeping stances upright and easy. Or, remain seated and only do the hand techniques in the form. You'd be surprised at how much better you can become if you can only concentrate on specific parts of the form. If your arm is what's broken, work on the leg techniques in the form. Work on deep stances, or wide stances. Work on the transition from one stance to the next. Work on beautiful technique. Worry about speed and power later. At first, focus on keeping flexible and on practicing those techniques that you can.

Read up on your martial art style as you recuperate. Learn about different styles—you might be able to use some of what you learn. Watch videos during those times when you would normally be working out— videos of martial arts masters in your field or even in another. Examine what they do, how they do it and why they do it.

As you ease your way back to class, try not to worry that you're not up to full speed. If possible, attend classes where you'll be allowed to participate at half speed.

When I broke my arm, I could still be do many techniques, but others were impossible. My partners were patient with me, however. If this is not the case at your school, you might want to be fully healed before returning to class. Practice half speed with a martial artist with whom you attend class, if you can, or have a non-martial artist friend work out with you. However, since it is considered dangerous to teach martial arts techniques except under controlled circumstances, don't teach them to your friend. In fact, most schools specifically prohibit you from teaching techniques to others unless you first receive the head instructor's permission. For this reason, if you are working out with a non-martial artist friend, confine your workouts to basic stretches and aerobic practice. If at any time, your injured area cramps, has sudden pain or otherwise responds negatively to the exercise, stop immediately and rest. If indicated, visit with your doctor.

Again, always pursue your fitness goals under the advice of a physician. With an injury begin by slowly and carefully using the affected limb. Limit difficult techniques, such as takedowns and the like. In the grappling arts, work on entering and balance breaking without actually throwing your partner or being thrown yourself.   This will help you to keep sharp without also re-injuring yourself. With a little thought and foresight, you can avoid injury, work out while pregnant and continue to grow as a martial artist even during physical rehabilitation.

8

Competition

One of the surprising pleasures of the martial arts is participating in competition. Some people are competitors in every sense of the word and thrive on the opportunities for competition that present themselves during the practice of the martial arts. And there are countless opportunities for competition in the martial arts. Many of these are informal competitions encountered in daily practice. Sometimes we compete against ourselves to improve our practice of techniques. One woman I know has a goal to learn each new form with fewer lessons than the last. This helps her be certain to concentrate and put her full attention on what her instructor is teaching her; it also makes her focus as she practices her forms so that she can do them without mistakes in the fewest number of attempts. She is a third degree black belt now, and the last very complex form she learned took her only two tries. Her instructor showed her and then she went through it twice, the second time without a mistake. I don't know how she'll improve upon that but I know she will try.

Sometimes we compete in friendly matches during class or perhaps we practice more formally for competition during practice by having "judges"—other students or instructors—look over our practice and evaluate us. But formal competition in the martial arts—the martial arts tournament—is a challenging, exhilarating and rewarding activity whether you win or lose.

Not being athletic myself, I had never had the chance to compete in sporting events. Sure, I competed in other ways—for grades and the like, but not in sports. Competing for grades is a very unsatisfying substitute for direct, head-to-head, one-on-one physical competition—but I didn't know this until I was twenty-seven years old. Although some women deeply dislike pitting their talents against others, it is a good way to learn just how much progress you are making in your practice. Besides, we all secretly wonder just how accomplished we really are, and tournament competition allows us to judge this, and it allows us to watch and compete against others whom we don't watch or compete against on a daily basis. I have learned some of my best techniques from watching others at tournaments and I have gained some valuable insights into my character while being soundly beaten by a much lower-ranking fighter.

So I have always felt that formal competition, win or lose, has its benefits, as long as we recognize that it is not the only thing in the martial arts world that matters and that it is not the only way we should judge our martial arts skills (although in some martial arts, such as Sambo, you are only promoted if you consistently win at tournaments!)

My instructor always called competition "good stress." He would say that you really couldn't know how you'd react in a stressful situation unless you actually made it a point to perform under stressful conditions. Being mugged, he would go on to say, was bad stress, but your body didn't act much differently under bad stress than it did under good stress. So you would be able to cope with the bad stress if you learned to cope with the good stress.

This is the question all martial artists ask themselves continually. Could I really defend myself? Am I really strong enough or skillful enough to prevent a personal attack? Performing in competition can help you gain more confidence, and can help you believe that the answer is yes—you are powerful enough to defend yourself. It doesn't matter whether you score a lot of points, win first place or don't place at all. What matters is confronting the fear and anxiety present and overcoming it.

And it takes practice. That's why it's a good idea to participate in tournaments whenever you can. Practicing your skills under stress helps give you confidence. Repeated practice increases your confidence. The first competition may make you so nervous that you fail. And that's okay. The next time, you will be more comfortable because you will know better what to expect.

Some people of course are blessed with a love of the pressure of competition. These are usually the same people who are blessed with great talent. For the rest of us, it helps to have as much ammunition as possible going in.

Since lack of experience or preparation can lead to frustrating and disappointing experiences, always try to obtain as much information as possible about the tournament before you go. The higher-ranking belts will often be good sources of information, since they will have more experience in competition than lower-ranking belts.

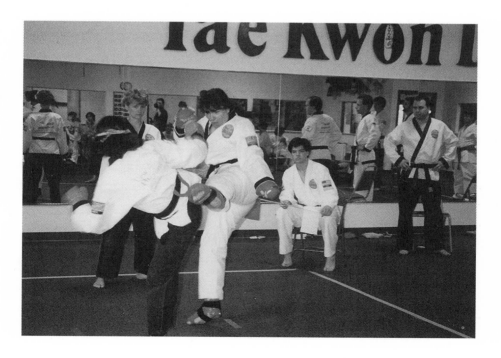

*Staging a tournament in your school can be excellent
practice for new competitors.*

Most martial arts instructors encourage their students to compete. Some arts, however, are not designed for competition. Traditional Aikido is one of these. Competition is thought to go against the spirit of some martial arts styles like this. Instructors of these styles say their martial art is not a sport subject to judges' decisions but rather a method of personal growth and spiritual development. This being the case, formal competition is thought to obstruct the appreciation and understanding of the true martial art. If this is the philosophy of your school, accept it as such. If you really do want to compete in tournament-style competitions, you will have to join a different school. Competing on your own when your instructor or school does not encourage tournament participation is considered dishonorable and is at the very minimum disrespectful to your instructor. You can take other opportunities to perform under stress. Perhaps your school does promotion testing, which requires that you perform your lessons in front of a judge or instructor. Or, you can ask higher belts to watch your techniques and correct them. In this way, you will be able to perform under stress, but the practice will be in a way that is acceptable to your instructor.

Most hard style schools—Karate and Tae Kwon Do, for instance—do actively encourage and sponsor martial arts competitions. These range from small in-school tournaments designed to give students a sense of what a tournament is about, to local competitions attended by a handful of area schools, to regional tournaments drawing from several states to, of course, national and international competition.

Starting small is not a bad idea at all, but many martial artists find themselves at regional tournaments on their first try because of the lack of local tournaments. This is somewhat intimidating but is still a good way to get your feet wet.

Choosing a Tournament

Most tournaments are by invitation only, although there are some that are open to anyone with a clean uniform. Invitational tournaments are simply those where your entire school is invited to attend by the host institution. You do not need a more specific invitation than that to attend. Ordinarily, these tournaments are arranged as one style only events, such as Tae Kwon Do only. Usually the martial arts schools participating are all well-known to each other, and may even by run by members of the same martial arts "family," —that is, instructors who learned together under one instructor who have gone on to open schools of their own. Occasionally, invitational tournaments will include similar styles; for instance, it is not uncommon for local or even regional tournaments to include both Karate schools and Tae Kwon Do schools. Some of the larger tournaments, primarily national or international in scope, invite all styles. Divisions are much more specific at these tournaments than at single style tournaments. The division is the group of people you will specifically compete against, since of course it would be unfair for seven-year-old kids to compete against adult men.

In single style tournaments, the divisions are usually pretty simple and straight forward. Each event is divided into adults' and children's divisions. Children's divisions are generally co-ed since weight and size in this group is completely unrelated to gender. The children's divisions are usually grouped according to age. The older teenagers are sometimes grouped into girls' and boys' divisions, but not very often. The adult groups are usually, although not always, divided into men's and women's divisions. There is often an executive division for older participants. The groups are then divided further by belt level, so that beginners, intermediate, and advanced practitioners all compete against people of roughly the same skill level. In bigger tournaments, if the divisions are still too large (and what is too large depends on the tournament organizers), groups will be further divided by light, middle and heavy weight, which, I was relieved to discover, is usually determined by height rather than weight. (Being short and fat meant I could nonetheless spar in the lightweight division—against other short, fat women!) Some tournaments have instructors' divisions so that instructors can compete without competing against their own students. Basically, then, at local and regional tournaments, a division will be something like "Black Belt Women's Sparring," which makes it simple. If you are a black belt woman who is competing in sparring, this is your division.

In bigger competitions, there are additional criteria used to create divisions, such as hard or soft style, weapons or empty-hand, and so on. This is slightly more confusing, but it means you can compete in a number of different categories—divisions—and gain a great deal of experience in this way. If, for instance, you practice Karate, you can compete in empty hand forms (kata) as well as weapons forms; in a smaller tournament, you would have only one opportunity to compete in a forms event.

Ordinarily, your school's instructor will post or announce tournament invitations or will let you know that an open tournament is being held. Usually, the instructor will only recommend those tournaments that fit with the school's overall philosophy. Suppose, for instance, your Karate school practices very light contact or no contact at all. Your instructor will not recommend full contact Karate tournaments in that case.

If you hear of a tournament you would be interested in watching, by all means go. But don't participate in a tournament without your instructor's permission. When you compete at a tournament, you represent your school—you are identified by your school. So your instructor might be hurt if he or she feels you have damaged the school's reputation by participating in a full contact tournament when he or she stresses no contact at school. Usually, black belts are given a little more latitude than lower belts— primarily because the instructor does not want a lower belt injured or even just discouraged by participating in inappropriate competitions.

Bare-knuckle, full contact, he-man type competitions are almost universally frowned on by martial arts instructors because they are unsafe forums that resemble street brawls and do not showcase martial arts techniques. In fact, such competitions have been outlawed in a number of states. The point of competition is to help you develop your confidence, improve your techniques and perform under stress. Coming home with three broken ribs and a bloody nose does not necessarily get you any closer to these goals.

Participating in safe, well-run tournament competitions is of course not the same as being confronted by a knife-wielding drugged-out attacker in a dark alley, but that is not the point. Competition will restrict the techniques you use, perhaps making groin and knee strikes off-limits, where in a real confrontation, nothing is off-limits. Truly dangerous techniques should be practiced under controlled conditions, using a heavy bag or with a partner who knows exactly what you are going to do. These techniques have no place in a tournament.

Choosing Your Events

Tournaments can have three basic types of contests: forms, sparring and breaking.

Forms competition is simply the judging of a person's performance of a form (kata or hyung). Participants select a form that best displays their talents and is appropriate to their belt level. Participants are evaluated on control, power and technique. In a contest including multiple styles, forms competition will be broken into soft styles, such as Wushu (Kung Fu) and hard styles, such as Karate, since it is difficult to compare a soft form to a hard form. Also, these groups will be further divided into weapons and empty hand forms, since again, it is difficult to compare a weapons form to an empty hand form. Sometimes musical forms competition is offered; here, artistic flair and harmony with the music are also evaluated. Some tournaments include pair or group forms, and in this case, the synchronicity of the participants is important.

In most cases, a panel of five judges score the form from 1 to 10, with the highest and lowest scores disregarded. Rarely does one who completes a form achieve less than a five.

In breaking contests, usually limited to Tae Kwon Do competitions and a few Karate tournaments, competitors are given a specified number of boards (usually one inch thick). The number usually varies by belt rank, with black belts having four or five boards to break. The competitor chooses the techniques with which she will try to break the boards. Sometimes tile or brick breaking is done.

If two competitors tie, the judges will select the technique used to break the tie-breaking boards. Five or sometimes six judges will award up to ten points, taking into consideration the difficulty of the technique, whether the technique was executed correctly and whether the board broke.

Sparring Competition

Judo Competition

Judo contests, called shiai, have very formal rules and procedures for sparring. The object in Judo is to throw the opponent to the ground, squarely on her back, and then pin her. The ring, a mat, allows about ten yards of room. A referee, two judges and a score keeper are required by Judo contest rules. The referee is in charge of the match, although the judges can disagree with his or her calls. A simple majority rules. At the end of a match, if the contestants are tied by points, decision is by judges' vote (hantei). The referee casts the deciding vote if the two judges cannot agree. Judo matches usually run from 6 to 10 minutes, with no rounds, although Olympic matches last 15 or 20 minutes. A full point (ippon) is awarded when an opponent is thrown forcefully onto his or her back, and he or she lands squarely on the mat. A full point is also awarded by immobilizing or locking the opponent for 30 seconds, or less if the opponent surrenders. If a contestant scores a full point, she wins the match and the match ends. Half points (waza-ari) are also awarded for throws that are not quite square or immobilizations that do not quite last 30 seconds. Two of these waza-ari can be added together to make ippon, one point. Two other scores are given: yuko, which is less than a half point, and koka, which is less than yuko. These two scores cannot be added to make a full point, but they are recorded and help judges arrive at decision at the end of a match, should neither contestant score a full point.

Penalties are assessed as points or partial points awarded to the non-penalized, so an individual can win a match merely because of the penalties given to her opponent. Depending on the severity of the rules infraction, the penalty can even be as much as a full point. Men, women, children, and teenagers all participate in different divisions.

Karate Competition

In Karate, sparring rules depend a great deal on the tournament organizers. Most Karate tournaments require no-contact sparring. Points are called when clean shots land extremely close to a target area; to land a kick or punch close but not on an opponent's body requires good control, and this is one of the ways in which contestants are judged. Those whose kicks and punches land or land too forcefully can be disqualified.

In traditional Japanese tournaments, if a technique is correctly executed and is not blocked, a point is awarded. Techniques that are not perfectly done or are partially blocked can earn half points. This one-point system is rarely used in the West.

Commonly, a point is awarded for a correct, clean technique, and no points are awarded for any technique that is not correctly executed; nor are points awarded for techniques that are blocked, whether partially or fully. A bout lasts two or three minutes, depending on the organizers. Whoever has accumulated the most points at the end of the round wins. A referee and a varying number of judges decide points and fouls. Competitors are usually given several warnings for rules infractions before being penalized. Once a foul has been called, usually after three warnings, the penalty is the loss of a point or the forfeit of the match. Fouls are usually assessed for contact that is too hard, or for kicks below the belt, although sometimes they are given for other infractions, such as turning away to avoid an attack instead of blocking or countering it, or stepping out of the ring to avoid an attack.

In most Karate tournaments, if a match ends in a tie, a sudden death overtime will be used; the first contestant to score a point wins. In a few tournaments, the winner is decided by who can break the most boards. A further sparring competition, the grand champion competition, is common to both Karate and Tae Kwon Do tournaments. In this contest, the winners of all black belt divisions compete to determine the single best competitor. Grand champion competitions are usually divided into men's grand champion and women's grand champion contests. Two rounds are required for a grand champion match, with a short rest between.

Semi-contact Karate has similar rules, but safety equipment is worn to protect the participants, and light contact is allowed. Such tournament sparring usually has two minute matches and determines the winner by the accumulated point system. Again, too much contact can lead to the deduction of points or the disqualification of a contestant. Professional Karate, or full-contact, is fought to the knockout. As in boxing, if no knockout occurs, a panel of judges decides the winner. In international competition, teams compete. Five people comprise a team, and the team with the most points accumulated wins. Tie-breaking matches consist of a match between each team's best fighter.

Kung Fu Competition

In Wushu (Kung Fu), sparring and forms competitions are conducted with and without weapons. Since there are so many styles and schools of Wushu, each tournament organizer specifies the rules for the tournament. These vary significantly.

Tae Kwon Do Competition

In Tae Kwon Do, matches are conducted as in Karate matches, with two or three minute rounds. Tae Kwon Do tournaments are always contact tournaments, and participants are usually required to wear protective gear. For a technique to count, it must be correctly performed, it must be unblocked, and it must cause a visible shock to the body of the opponent. Hand techniques to the head are not usually allowed, although kicks to the head are accepted in many tournaments. A center ring judge, who acts as a referee, and four corner judges (the ring is actually a square) determine the scoring in a match. A majority of judges must see the point and agree that it counts. In some competitions, a panel of judges (as many as five plus the center ring judge) will score the match independently and the winner will be determined by decision. Fouls are called for stepping out of bounds on purpose, for using throws or takedowns, for avoiding the fight and other infringements. These result in the penalty of a full or half point deduction. In some tournaments, foot techniques earn higher scores than hand techniques; jumping techniques are scored higher than standing techniques; a kick to the head is worth more than one to the body.

Aikido Competition

In Aikido, competition is not traditionally allowed, but some schools do participate in competition. Three kinds of sparring contests occur: ninin-dori, in which one contestant spars against two attackers; tanto-randori, in which an empty-handed contestant spars against an armed attacker; and randori-kyoghi, in which two empty handed participants try to score against each other with properly applied techniques.

Preparing for Competition

These are simply the general guidelines for tournament competition. Specific rules for tournaments will vary according to the organizers. Know the rules before you enter, and be certain you understand them before you participate.

Of course, the invitation or announcement will usually provide most of the rules information. If you have difficulty deciphering this, don't hesitate to ask your instructor or the tournament's organizers. Be aware, however, that tournaments are fluid events. It pays to be flexible. Perhaps you are an older woman and you plan to enter the executive division, which the rules say is for people 35 and over. Sometimes, especially in women's competition at the local and regional level, there will only be a few women who register for this division, so the division will be cancelled, and you'll be expected to join the regular women's division, in which case all those flexible 18-year-olds will be showing off. This is okay. Maturity has its rewards, not least of which is patience and a good attitude. Or, instead of combining the women's executive division with the regular women's division, the organizers might combine the women's executive division with the men's executive division. Now, if you have followed my advice and sparred lots of men, this turn of events will leave you tranquil. Again, it simply pays to be aware that divisions can change (their boundaries are very fluid sometimes), and that specific rules can change.

In breaking competition, most Tae Kwon Do tournaments allow black belts four boards. I participated in a tournament in which more people registered at the door than expected, and the organizers did not have a sufficient number of boards. So black belts were asked to use three boards. This, you may say, is not really a big deal since it is in fact easier to break three boards than four, but it rattled quite a number of the contestants who had practiced one way of breaking their boards—and one way only!—and when they had to change, they became angry and frustrated. Those who simply accepted the change, rethought their strategy, and tried to show themselves to the best advantage using only three boards were of course the contestants who won.

Again, because there are far fewer women who practice the martial arts than there are men, we need to be a little more flexible than they do, and what works for them may not work exactly right for us. For instance, when preparing for a tournament, men usually practice sparring with those at their own level or higher. At a tournament, there are always a vast number of male competitors, and therefore they usually have more divisions, and more people in their divisions than women do. In fact, I have never attended a tournament with the numbers of men and women being anywhere close to equivalent. So when men practice sparring only others at their level, they are certain to put this experience to good practice at the tournament. This is always a good idea, but it doesn't prepare you for everything. As a newly-minted brown belt, I once entered a tournament in which only five color belt (non-black belt) women participated. Instead of dividing us into lower and higher belt groups as is usually done, the organizers had all of us spar each other. For the final match, I had an orange belt as an opponent. An orange belt in Tae Kwon Do is still quite a beginner; she had been practicing a little over four months. I had been at it much longer. To even the field, the judges agreed to give her two points at the start; the first one of us to five would win. I, of course, was supremely confident that I would win, but I was also concerned about tournament sparring someone so inexperienced. Guess what? The orange belt won. I learned a great deal—which meant that in a way I had won, too. But it was a little embarrassing.

I learned, of course, not to underestimate an opponent, and I learned that patronizing someone with less experience was wrong. There was no need for me to beat her up just to demonstrate my fighting prowess, but I could have sparred her appropriately by using only those techniques that an orange belt would know and by being certain to practice good control. These are things I do all the time when sparring in all belt classes to make it interesting. But I never made the connection to tournament sparring. I simply felt uncomfortable trying to beat someone with so little experience, so I didn't even try to win.

Still, it is never going to be quite fair to anyone when two vastly different skill levels compete, which is one of the reasons why your tournament focus shouldn't be just on winning. In my match with the orange belt, she had to overcome her intimidation. If you see a much higher ranking opponent across the ring from you, it doesn't matter how confident you are, you will still be unsettled. I was once the only female black belt competitor in a local tournament, so the organizer tossed me in with the guys—and I am not the only woman who has had this happen. A friend of mine practices a form of Karate that is no-holds-barred; not only is she the only woman in her school, but she is consistently the only woman who competes in this style of Karate. Since we both are accustomed to practicing with men all the time, such events are not completely unnerving, but it is a little daunting to compete against men in tournament, because in contrast to when they are competing against other men, who might have superior skills or have been at it longer (or were bigger or any one of a number of excuses), a man competing in tournament against a woman feels his very manhood is at stake if he loses, and so instead of a normal person facing you across the ring, you get an aggressive lunatic.

To prepare for competition, you must practice according to the published rules of the tournament. But you must also be prepared for otherwise unexpected changes in those rules. If for instance, the tournament rules say that the target area is the chest from the shoulders to the waist, then your high roundhouse kick should be mothballed for a while, even though you would ordinarily use it during sparring practice. This sort of practice is essential, even if your partners continue to do high roundhouse kicks to the head. However, I have attended tournaments where rules such as this were published, and then the contestants prevailed upon the organizers to change the rules to allow kicks to the head. So you can't forget how to use that high roundhouse kick; you simply need to practice without it for a while. If you learn that after all you will be able to use that kick, it should still be there for you.

In sparring I have always relied a great deal on hand techniques. I do many punches to the middle and in fact practice boxing to improve my punching. My favorite technique to the high section is not a kick, it is a backfist to the temple. It is my favorite because as a hand technique it is faster than a foot technique, and since most people don't keep their heads covered, it actually lands a lot. But in Tae Kwon Do tournaments, punches aren't really "seen" by the judges—though a good clean punch is worth a point, the judges are really looking for kicks more than anything else. So for me to do a middle punch that scores a point, my opponent must be wide, wide open, I have to stick my punch, kihop very loudly to get everyone's attention, and hold my position until a judge eventually realizes that I have landed a blow, and yells, "point!" Usually, however, by this time my opponent has dropped an ax kick on my head, and it's her technique that the judges see, so she gets the point. Or, since she has scored on a high target area, two points. So I am at a disadvantage in a tournament unless I practice several weeks ahead of time by not using middle punches—or, if I use them, to know they are not to score points but as lead-ins for other techniques, such as an ax kick.

In addition, most Tae Kwon Do tournaments do not allow hand techniques to the head, so the backfist to the temple that I rely on will not score any points. In fact, it will get me into trouble, because if I use an illegal technique—and if the tournament organizers say no hand techniques to the head then my backfist to the temple is an illegal technique—I can be warned, lose points, and even be disqualified from the match or the entire tournament. If I do it often enough, the organizers will specifically not invite me back. So it is then imperative that I practice sparring without using my backfist at all, which, since it is so automatic, can be difficult to quit using. But this type of practice is useful in other ways as well. It forces me to think of other techniques to use when I see an opening for a backfist. And having more than one technique ready would serve me well in a confrontation—especially, let us imagine, if I have injured my hand already. I would not be inclined to use it further, and I might not be able to do the technique with as much power as usual. By practicing according to the tournament rules, you'll be much more comfortable and confident come competition time.

I once won my division relying on all those punches to the middle, but it was actually a Karate tournament, not a Tae Kwon Do tournament (most Karate schools emphasize hand techniques, whereas Tae Kwon Do schools emphasize foot techniques). In this case, my tendencies paid off—but I also benefitted from knowing the rules ahead of time and practicing my sparring according to the rules, which favored punches. Of course, my Tae Kwon Do colleagues gave me no end of grief for winning a division in a Karate tournament, but then they had all participated too and were just jealous because their high kicks to the head didn't count.

As you prepare for competition, encourage other school members to imitate the tournament atmosphere. If you stay after class to practice your form, ask a higher ranking belt to judge your performance. Doing a form under the watchful gaze of a higher ranking student can be a bit nerve-wracking. As you practice sparring, ask the instructor if he or she would be willing to call out points as he or she sees them, or have a group of tournament-goers meet before or after class, with the instructor's permission, and set up a ring with judges. Practice sparring in a ring in front of judges. Sometimes you'll score a point but the judges won't see it, or not enough judges will see it (you need a majority) and if you let that frustrate you, you won't be able to win. You will be flustered, angry or resentful, none of which will keep your attention focused where it should be.

Tournament sparring usually calls for a break when a point has been called. The center ring judge, hearing a corner judge yell "point!" will separate the contestants, and stop the sparring. The center ring judge will then ask how many corner judges saw a point. If a sufficient number did, then a point will be awarded. The official scorekeeper must always wait for the specific directive of the center ring judge. Usually time keeps running while points are decided, but sometimes it does not. This is important to know, because a two-minute bout in which time keeps running while points are decided actually affords far fewer scoring opportunities than the two-minute bout in which time is stopped whenever tournament action stops.

Since practice sparring is usually continuous, the way action is stopped during a tournament match can really interfere with your strategy, especially if you use a countering style of sparring. In this case, the opponent may land the first blow, which you would usually then counter. But if the action is stopped while the judges decide if that first blow counted for a point, that great countering technique you had planned won't get you anywhere. It doesn't matter what the judges decision is—point or not, you go back to your starting position and begin again. Thus, it is important to practice stopping a match during sparring. You might work with a partner and just informally pause and step back to acknowledge when your partner has landed a technique that might be considered a point. If your partner will do the same whenever you execute a technique that might be called a point, both of you will improve your tournament sparring skills.

In this type of competition, you always know how many points you and your opponent have. This can be frustrating when your opponent is several points ahead of you. If you are several points ahead of her, it may cause you to lay back, or enter a prevent defense, which may win football games but does not win sparring matches. If you practice sparring for points, you'll learn to anticipate and overcome your reactions and tendencies before you enter the tournament ring.

One woman I work out with only gets more aggressive if her opponent is outscoring her. In a way she is almost better off if she gets behind in a match. The drawback is that a two-minute match is actually pretty short and she might simply not have the opportunity to gain back the points and win. Another woman finds this discouraging and so tries to jump out ahead from the very beginning by aggressively charging after that first point, while her opponent might be still just feeling her out. This works to her advantage sometimes, because such an offense can be overwhelming, but a good competitor can stop her charge and take advantage of it. For myself, I have a tendency to be aggressive without being aware of how many points are being scored on me. I am only ever worried about how many points I am scoring. This disregard for the opponent's performance has its advantages, but also its drawbacks. I don't often change my strategy to accommodate for an opponent who is expecting a front kick-middle punch-crescent kick combination. Instead, I always just go ahead and fire it off, never mind if I immediately find a reverse kick in my stomach. This sort of thing helps me to lose matches I should otherwise win. So I have to practice point sparring differently from other people. I actually need a coach to stop me and remind me that I am behind in points with thirty seconds left, so I need to be more defensive and let the opening come to me instead of trying to charge ahead and make the opening happen, getting nailed for another point in the process.

None of these approaches is necessarily right or wrong, but being aware of the potential drawbacks of your sparring tendencies can be helpful.

Sometimes sparring matches are continuous, however, with the judges scoring independently. This is an equally difficult type of match to fight, but for different reasons. First of all, you never know the score, so you have no idea of how aggressive you need to be. You have no idea what types of techniques the judges are seeing and counting, so you can't rearrange your strategy to account for that. It is difficult enough to spar when you know how you are doing, but it is much more difficult—and disconcerting—when you have no idea how the judges think you are doing.

The best way to spar a continuous independently judged matched is to yell loud, stick your kicks and punches and block aggressively so that no one will think that front kick snuck through your guard.

Be certain to talk to veteran tournament-goers, including people who have been to the specific tournament you are planning to participate in and those who just have lots of tournament experience in general. They can help you understand what the judges are looking for. For instance, in men's breaking competition, the judges tend to look for techniques of a high degree of difficulty, since of the twenty or so men competing in the division, at least half will break all their boards on the first try, and there are only three places to award. So the judges must determine which of these are worthy of placing. Real power—for instance, kicking through four boards at once—is admired, while a kick through two boards is not considered that impressive in men's board breaking. Very technical performances are also admired; I once watched a competitor break a board in half with a jumping spinning heel kick, and then, without setting down, break the half board remaining in the holder's hand with another jump spinning heel kick. The remaining three boards he broke all at once with a ridge hand speed break. Since these techniques required finesse, accuracy and great confidence, the judges awarded him the first place honors. Of course, part of the judges' appreciation was that they hadn't seen this exact combination tried before, so part of its appeal was unique. The next year at the same tournament, a number of competitors were doing similar techniques, so it had lost some of its charm.

On the other hand, since women's divisions are smaller, and women in general have more difficulty breaking boards because they usually can't just power their way through, as men can, the guiding principle, so often repeated that it has become a mantra among us, is simply, break the boards, all of them, on the first try. In a division with five women competing, perhaps two of them will break all their boards on the first try; a third might break some on the first try and some on the second try. These competitors will win first, second and third place. So the emphasis is slightly different. If "break the boards" is rule number one, then "break them with power" is rule number two. Since most of the judges will be men, they like to see men-type things, such as punching and breaking more than one board at a time. A jump reverse kick through two boards followed by a punch through two boards will win a women's board breaking competition sooner than four individual breaks will.

Of course, since the number one rule is to break all the boards on the first try, unless I am supremely confident of my power techniques, I need to rely instead on speed techniques, which are admired because of their high degree of difficulty. However, I have seen very simple combinations win women's breaking: a side kick, front kick, reverse kick and elbow smash once won first place in black belt women's division even though all of these techniques are the very first techniques taught to Tae Kwon Do practitioners. The practitioner won simply because all the boards broke the first time. Practice board breaks several times before a tournament; remember that adrenaline will throw you off. I always kick higher at tournaments than during tests or practice, so even though it kills me to do it, I make the holders keep the boards about six inches higher than I think I am going to kick because that is exactly where my kick is going to land. But I never feel entirely comfortable about this until after the boards break.

But again, winning isn't everything. I once attempted a jump reverse kick through four boards at a tournament. None of the judges—or even participants—had ever seen a woman even try this (they thought I was kidding at first). I simply wanted to see if I could do it; I also knew my competitors at board breaking—they never missed. Whereas I do sometimes miss. Perhaps my ulterior motive was simply to try and break all the boards at one time so I wouldn't be out there banging on boards for half an hour. At any rate, I gave it two good tries, the maximum number of tries allowed at this tournament, failed to break any boards, bowed out to the judges and lost the competition. Afterward, however, I heard only good things. The two people who placed first and second, I was told, always do the same breaks. How can they get better if they keep doing the same breaks over and over? Well, I said, you may not get better, but you do in fact win tournaments that way. Some people congratulated me simply for trying. One of my male friends went ahead and tried the same break just because I had. He didn't break at that tournament but he did at a later one, and he won the competition with a technique that he would never otherwise have tried. One of the judges said, "I was hoping you could do it. I know you can do it." I am not ordinarily one who inspires that much belief. Let it be said, however, that trying is everything: in my black belt test I broke three boards with a jump reverse kick on the first try even though I had never done it before just because I thought I could.

Talking approaches over with more experienced tournament competitors can help you relax and enjoy a rewarding experience. When I first started competing, I was accustomed to practicing on a carpeted floor. The first tournament I attended was in a gym with hardwood floors. This made footwork much different. Wet spots were slippery instead of just wet, and my sweating feet stuck to the floor. Pivoting was impossible to do in one fluid movement. Later, I participated in a tournament held on a padded floor. The floor covering was actually a wall-to-wall mat with a foam rubber-like surface. My feet sank into the floor, making turns and pivoting difficult, unless I really picked up my feet and exaggerated every movement. I nearly wrecked my hips forever, not to mention my knees, on that horrible surface. Needless to say, those participants who were accustomed to using mats had a much easier time of it. Had I known, or even thought about the difference in flooring, I might have, at the very minimum gotten to the site earlier in the day to practice my form. The site might also influence the form you select. Limited space requires a different approach than lots of space. Try to find out everything you can from the availability of lockers and changing rooms to the number of rings.

So understand the site, see it if possible, know the rules and consult with others who have been there and done that, and remember that even if you don't take away a trophy, you'll take away some excellent lessons.

9

Choosing a School

With the right attitude, plus persistence and a clear understanding of herself and her body, any woman can become a better martial artist, even an exceptional martial artist. Being aware of potential injuries can help you avoid disrupting your training. Capitalizing on your strengths will boost your self-confidence and improve your technical and fighting skills. But one of the most important ways you can help yourself is to choose a female-friendly, supportive school. If you are just thinking about joining a martial arts school, or if you already belong to one but don't think it is giving you what you need, knowing how to choose a martial arts school can help you make the right decision.

How to choose a martial arts school

Most people put very little thought into choosing a martial arts school. They go to the nearest one or the cheapest one, because, unfortunately, that's how people make most decisions. But when it comes to choosing a martial arts school, this practice can be dangerous and, over time, can prove very costly. Choosing the right martial arts school is important not only for safety and cost, but because many students drop out simply because they chose the wrong school. For women, finding a female-friendly school is essential. To prevent wasted time and money, a well-informed decision should be made. However, most people know very little about the martial arts when they begin; for this reason, they do not know what they should look for in a school. Time invested in determining which school is right for you will pay off in the long run. That's where this information will help you.

Obviously, your choices are limited by the kinds of schools that are within a reasonable distance of your home, but other than that, how do you choose the right school? There are several factors you will have to consider. Choosing a martial arts style and setting martial arts goals are personal decisions you will have to make. You will also have to find a school that has good teachers, and is in good condition with appropriate equipment. You will have to decide what size school is best for you. You will need to make sure that other students are similar to you, or you may not fit in well. You will need to check references, figure costs and interview the head instructor. How much weight you give each element in the decision is up to you, but all these factors should be considered.

The first step is to decide which martial arts style appeals to you most. Chapter One discussed the various styles most commonly available to people; now is the time for a little homework.

Choosing a martial arts style

Which style appeals to you most? Check your phone directory to see what kinds of schools are listed there. You might be surprised at the number of possibilities within a reasonable distance. Once you know what's available, you have to decide: Would you rather punch and kick your way to better health, or would you prefer to grapple your way there? The young and flexible might choose a style that emphasizes high kicks, speed and power. This shouldn't stop a less young and less flexible individual from choosing such a style, but she should be aware that other styles might complement her needs better. Someone with arthritis or hip problems might have difficulty obtaining the flexibility needed for Tae Kwon Do; therefore, Aikido might be more suitable. T'ai Chi is an excellent choice for those who are older or have physical problems that might impede their ability to do a lot of striking techniques. Try to watch practitioners from the various styles before making a choice. Try not to let what you've seen on television or in the movies influence your decision too much. Ask yourself, as you watch, if you could actually imagine yourself performing the techniques that you see. This doesn't mean that you have to be able to do those techniques now; one of the great benefits of the martial arts is learning how to do things you didn't know you could do. Still, it should be within the realm of possibility for you.

Be sure to stop by several training halls (schools, also known as "dojo" or "dojang") and watch classes. It is important to find a school that is within reasonable distance from your home; you are more likely to continue attending if getting there isn't a burden. Therefore, driving (or walking or taking the bus) to the school will help you see which schools are easiest to get to. Also, try not to make your decision until you've seen students from different schools in action. In the striking styles, such as Tae Kwon Do and Karate, the physical contact allowed during sparring varies. Some schools are no-contact schools, so while you risk less injury, the fighting situation does not resemble reality very closely. Some school allow light contact, which helps you to judge the distance between you and your opponent better, and also helps you develop good control. Some schools encourage medium or heavy contact, which most closely resembles the fighting situations in which you might find yourself, but also increases the risk of injury. You need to decide what amount of contact is right for you. Ask the head instructor to describe the amount of contact that is allowed; if possible, ask some students as well, because people have different opinions about what light, medium and heavy contact are.

Some schools divide classes by age into "adult" and "child" classes, or by rank such as "white through orange belt" and "green belt and above." Some schools offer classes for women only, so they can learn self-defense techniques, but this has limited usefulness. By this I mean your partners will be women, who do tend to be less physically strong than men; demonstrating that you can get away from a five foot three, one hundred and ten pound woman is not the same as demonstrating that you can get away from a six foot two, two hundred pound man. As a woman, it is the latter you will most likely have to worry about. On the other hand, such classes can make a woman feel more comfortable with the martial arts. Once she is more confident of her skills, she can join coed classes. Women's classes may also make you feel less self-conscious. Another benefit is that instructors and participants are willing to discuss specific threats to women.

Be sure to watch a class that most closely corresponds to the class you would be attending (ie, watch adult classes if you are an adult; how children are taught may have nothing to do with how adults are taught.)

Sometimes a city will have several schools that teach the same style. Most likely, each school emphasizes different aspects of the style. If this is the case, other factors besides martial art style are important. You will have to weigh each element and decide which ones are most important to you.

Determining your martial arts goals

As you decide on the style you think is most suitable, ask yourself what your martial arts goals are. At this point, it may be difficult for you to know. Without prior experience, it is hard to set goals. The first thing to consider is how much time you will be able to spend at it. The serious martial artist who plans to work out two hours a day six days a week desires something different from an individual who plans to use martial arts as a form of exercise twice a week. These people will probably want to attend different schools.

Or perhaps you have always been interested in the martial arts and you really want to immerse yourself in the culture and philosophy of the art as well as pay attention to the physical component. You will have different needs from someone who is interested in concentrating on the sport aspect.

If you decide you really want to earn a black belt and become proficient at tournament sparring, more power to you. The key is to just be certain that you are in the right school. For instance, a university-sponsored or parks-and-recreation Karate class that meets twice a week for two months, then has a break, then meets a few weeks, then has semester break, then meets with a lot of new students, then breaks, may not be the ideal choice, though it may be the cheapest. On the other hand, for someone whose goals are less lofty, the cheaper, more convenient choice might be the best.

Keep in mind that some schools do not emphasize competition, and so they will not be invited to nor will they compete in tournaments. This means you won't either, which may or may not hurt your feelings. If you are interested in the sport aspect of martial arts, check out the trophies in the training hall. If there are none, you'll know that tournaments are not important. If there are lots, then tournaments are important to the school, though that doesn't necessarily mean anything about the students' skills or the instructor's expertise. It may mean that they participate in lots of small local and regional tournaments. This is not necessarily bad; you may want to start small and work your way up. Ask the school's head instructor.

Perhaps your goal is to learn excellent self-defense skills while working on your fitness level. You will want to choose a school that can provide a lot of practical self-defense techniques, or one that offers special self-defense classes. Or perhaps you are really interested in focusing on fitness and conditioning. You will want to choose the school with killer workouts. It is becoming more and more common for fitness centers to include martial arts classes along with aerobics and weight lifting. This might certainly be a good choice for someone interested in all-around fitness, but evaluate such martial arts schools carefully, to be certain they are staffed and run by well-trained martial artists.

There's no reason your martial arts goals can't change over time. Plenty of people join the martial arts to improve fitness and find the driving urge to earn a black belt. Some people who are only motivated by the thought of attaining a black belt may never make it past the first few months of training—or may quit practicing when they reach black belt level.

Still, identifying your martial arts goals, even if they are vague at the beginning, can help you choose the right school. It also gets you into the habit of goal setting, which is an important part of martial arts training.

Determining the quality of teaching

Choosing a school with good teachers is the most crucial element of all, but it is the most often overlooked or misunderstood. The head instructor sets the tone for the school, so you will want to meet with him or her before making a decision. There may be assistant instructors, so be sure you watch them in action, too. You may not have the same opinion of all the teachers in the school, but you should have a very favorable opinion of them as a group. Be aware, though, that just one assistant instructor who drives you nuts can become a problem in the long run. Don't ignore what could become a difficult situation; on the other hand, don't make too much of a simple difference in personality. It is a good idea to choose a school that has at least a few female instructors and several female black belts.

The use of assistant instructors doesn't necessarily mean anything good or bad about a school, but the head instructor should also be actively teaching. If he or she teaches only infrequently or teaches only upper belts, you aren't going to get what you're going to pay for. You can simply ask how often the head instructor teaches; if you don't get a straight answer, that's a good warning sign.

A good martial arts instructor will insist on a certain amount of respect and courtesy. This is not related to ego; it is merely the best way to enforce discipline, which is one of the elements of the martial arts that is most difficult to maintain in a school. A good martial arts teacher takes his or her teaching and art very seriously. If everyone is having a lot of fun, they probably aren't working hard enough. This doesn't mean you can't ever crack a smile. A good teacher will motivate students to work harder, but without ridicule. Be aware of nuances. Do men and women work together or are they segregated? In a martial arts class, the less attention paid to gender, the better. Schools that separate participants by gender, instead of something pertinent, such as age, height or skill level, are doing both men and women a disservice.

As you observe a class, watch the instructor. Does the instructor move around the room, correcting the students' techniques? The instructor should demonstrate a technique and explain it, but he or she should also fix incorrect techniques that students display. Often, the instructor will describe what he or she is correcting on one student so that all students can hear. This is not meant to embarrass anyone; it is considered a good method of teaching more than one person at a time, since most students make similar mistakes in technique.

A good martial arts instructor does not yell; he or she is able to command attention without doing so. But a good instructor might, for no apparent reason, assign everyone twenty knuckle pushups. This is simply a fact of martial arts training. Be aware that a martial arts instructor is not like your high school science teacher. A martial arts instructor is training you to fight. You will be expected to improve your physical conditioning, to give your best effort, to work your hardest. Often, the instructor will set physical challenges for you that he or she expects you to meet. For instance, you might be told to hold a kick for one full minute. Or you might be told to concentrate on a target for several minutes without moving your eyes. These challenges improve your skills and also contribute to your strength, flexibility and discipline. Still, if your instinct or experience tells you that an instructor is more harmful than helpful, you will want to stay away. A good teacher will push you to your limits but not beyond; a good teacher may make you sore but should never make you hurt.

Checking the condition of the school

When you visit the training hall, try not to let fancy trappings lure you or worn carpet dissuade you. Carpet gets easily worn out during martial arts practice and mirrors are easily broken, but they are extremely expensive to replace. Very few martial arts schools turn large enough profits to look brand new all the time. You want to beware of those schools that do turn large profits; you will be paying for them. Also, unnecessary luxuries will come out of your pocket as well. Training costs are high enough without adding on special lighting or oak panelled waiting rooms. On the other hand, the training hall should always be clean and neat, which shows pride and respect. The locker room facilities should be adequate. You will never find a Jacuzzi in a training hall. Or almost never. Such facilities should be neat and clean. A shower is nice and so are lockers, but a toilet and shelves will do. If there is no separate women's locker room, that should tell you a lot about a school.

Check out the equipment. At the minimum, there should be mirrors (so that you can see what you are doing), a heavy bag (for practicing full power kicks and punches), kicking targets (in schools that kick), and carpet or mats (mats are especially important for grappling schools). All equipment should be in good shape. The heavy bag, while it may be removable, should have secure ceiling mountings. A water fountain is a nice extra, but the lack of one can be overcome be bringing a water bottle with you.

The key here is not to expect the same environment as you might find at the brand new gym that just opened up out in the suburbs, with shiny new bench presses. A training hall is simply a big room where students get together to work out. Beyond that, you want to make sure any extras are worth paying for.

Choosing the right size of school

Determining what size of school is right for you can be a difficult part of the decision making process. As in any other school, size has advantages and disadvantages.

When watching the class, ask yourself if there seems to be enough room for everyone to perform the techniques. If students are stumbling into each other, that simply means a frustrating experience awaits. But before ruling out the school entirely, you may want to find out why it's so crowded. It can mean you've found a good school, but of course it can also mean you'll have difficulty getting a good work out and receiving personal attention. Remember, however, that seeing one large class does not mean all classes are large. Perhaps the school has outgrown its present location, but the head instructor has plans to change locations soon. A successful martial arts school is often measured by size; an instructor who can build a large school and retain students is usually a good one. However, some perfectly mediocre and even bad schools are big, often because they have tapped into a certain aspect of the martial arts that appeals to people.

You can determine the size of the school by asking the head instructor how many students are active; asking for the average class size is also a good idea. In most cities and towns, more than 150 students is considered very large. Around 100 to 125 students is considered big; many instructors feel they have succeeded when they have this many active students. Fifty to 100 is a pretty successful medium-sized school. Under fifty is usually considered small. Small isn't necessarily bad. A smaller school may mean you get more individual attention. But again, you have to know why the school is small. Has it just started? Is the instructor deliberately keeping it small? Or does the instructor aggravate students and drive them off? It can be exciting to start with a newer school; the instructors are still very enthusiastic about what they are doing and you'll get a great deal of individual attention. Of course, you'll have to be prepared for the time to come when the school is larger and more successful. You may have to give up some of that special attention.

Working with an instructor who deliberately keeps his or her school small can also be rewarding. Some martial arts instructors have full time day jobs, since being a martial arts instructor is an extremely precarious way to make a living. Such martial arts instructors can be quite skilled and you can learn much from them. However, if you are not the instructor's primary business and computer programming is, you may find yourself losing out to computer programming.

A larger school has more facilities available, but assistant instructors will teach much of the time. Still, a larger school provides you with many different partners to work with, all of whom have different skills and aptitudes. This can challenge and improve you. Ultimately, choosing the size of school is up to you. You must decide what makes you more comfortable.

Learning about formality and structure

Each martial arts style and school has a different degree of structure and formality. For some people, much formality and structure is annoying and interferes with their learning and ability to improve. Such students will want to choose a less formal school. Other students, however, enjoy a structured, formal approach. They know what to expect and can mentally prepare themselves for each class. These students thrive in more highly structured environments.

As you observe a class, ask yourself if the students seem courteous to each other and to the instructor. Do instructors assist and correct techniques, or do they merely call out commands? Do children run around or are they expected to practice quietly? No matter what level of structure and formality you prefer, you should be able to expect other students to be courteous and under control.

Are you comfortable with the level of discipline you see? Some schools emphasize structure and formality more than others. How much structure do you want? The more traditional schools will offer the most structure; these are schools that are most likely to emphasize the entire martial arts experience, not just one aspect of it. Structure means that all classes follow similar approaches. For instance, a traditionally structured Tae Kwon Do class begins with the students lining up and performing punching and kicking drills. Then, basic movements are reviewed. Next, combinations of kicks are performed. The first half of class ends with forms practice; each student reviews several rank-specific forms. The second half of class consists of practicing step sparring, demonstrating power kicks and working on freestyle sparring. Students then line up again and perform some cool-down calisthenics.

Each time a student comes to class, he or she can expect a similar structure, with occasional variations to keep the students alert, especially at the more advanced levels. Such a highly structured environment might appeal to you. Or it might drive you crazy.

Still, it is important for there to be some consistency between classes. If possible, watch more than one class so that you can see the consistency between classes. Do different instructors run things differently? How differently? You do not want to be at the mercy of every instructor's whim, or you'll never learn what you need to know.

The classes should be well-supervised. Ask if an instructor is always available, watching and directing the class. Observe. Is the instructor yelling or teaching? You may not understand everything that you see, but you should be sure that the environment seems appropriate to you.

The level of formality in a school is mostly a matter of how much courtesy is expected of each student. Common sense will tell you that no matter what, students should be polite to each other. Beyond that, schools vary considerably in their levels of formality.

Some very formal schools expect students to bow when entering and leaving the training hall. This is merely a courtesy, a sign of respect, and is not religious in any way. Students may be expected to bow to instructors or other, higher-ranking students. Students may be expected to refer to black belts as "Mr. Smith" and "Ms. Jones" and to respond to directives with "yes, sir" or "yes, ma'am." While a student may be uncomfortable or forgetful at first, such formality makes the training hall a more pleasant, peaceful place. However, if such formality intimidates you or provokes a bad reaction, you will want to find a more casual school.

Checking similarities to other students

Nothing can be more disheartening than to belong to a school whose members are completely different from you. By this, I do not mean race or ethnic differences, but age and physical differences. If you are fifty years old and all those around you are eighteen, you will find yourself discouraged and frustrated by the experience, as anyone who has ever been surrounded by eighteen-year-olds can tell you. As you watch classes, look at the participants. Are any your age? It doesn't have to be a majority or even a lot. A few will do. As a woman, you should be certain that other women attend classes. Much as you may wish to destroy sexist stereotypes, you probably don't want to find yourself being the first female student in a traditionally all-male school. Unless of course you do want to do this; more power to you. Most schools are eager to work with both male and female students, so this is usually not a problem, but do check to make sure a number of other women work out at the school you are thinking of joining.

As you watch the students, ask yourself if you think you would fit in or if you would be intimidated by the energy, endurance and superb condition of everyone. This isn't necessarily bad, but if it only intimidates you and doesn't motivate you, it will probably lead to an unpleasant experience. You should feel a little impressed but not overwhelmed (unless you are watching a class for black belts only or something very advanced). If your family intends to join, or if you are looking at schools for your child as well, be certain that the school is family-oriented. Some schools train only adults; others teach both adults and children.

What is the atmosphere? Friendly? Very serious? Casual? For most martial artists, a friendly but formal atmosphere is optimal. It allows you to get the maximum benefit from your efforts, but you should also be able to meet people and talk to them. One of the pleasures of martial arts training is the social element, so unless you already have way too much social life, choose the school where students linger after class to talk.

You may not feel comfortable in any training hall right away, especially if you are unused to fighting, don't watch boxing and have never heard of Bruce Lee, but some halls will naturally seem to suit you better than others.

Finding and checking references

Once you have visited the various schools in your area and are ready to narrow your choices, ask other people for recommendations. You will be surprised at how many people participate in the martial arts. Ask friends and work associates if they have heard anything good or bad about the school. Be careful when judging the answers, though. If a friend heard a rumor from another friend's cousin, the information may not be reliable, but if the friend herself had a personal experience, the information can be very valuable. Current students will usually have only good things to say, but you can ask anyway. Sometimes they will provide you with important pieces of information about the school.

Next, find out if the school is well established. How long has it been in business? Longer usually means better; it means the owner/head instructor is competent enough to attract and keep students and it means that injuries are under control, which is extremely important. On the other hand, there are benefits to starting with a new school, but you should be aware that it is a new school. Check also with the area Better Business Bureau and the local Chamber of Commerce to make sure no complaints have been filed.

Figuring cost

One of the most important questions you'll ask is "How much does it cost?" Most martial arts schools don't make a lot of profit; a little comparison shopping should show you if someone is way out of line. Most martial artists feel that cost should be only a small part of the decision you make, and that is true. But cost is important, because you only have so much money, so you'd better spend it wisely. Be aware of the usual salesperson techniques. Martial arts sales are growing in sophistication and with that comes the usual hard-sell, sign up now-or-never approaches that used-car salespeople so admire. Avoid such schools if at all possible.

Unlike other activities, where you might pay by the hour or the number of classes, most martial arts schools operate by tuition. For a certain tuition, you attend however many classes you wish. Almost all schools offer two or three year plans where you pay all the tuition up front. In return, you get a discount. This is not a bad program, but you should never ever sign up for that much time and money until you know that you will continue in your martial arts training. Make certain that you like the style you have chosen and the school you have selected before committing a great deal of money to it. Most schools have introductory offers, where you can pay for a trial period of sixty days or three months. After that time, you can choose the two or three year program if you want. Some programs allow you to pay monthly; others ask that you pay for one full year ahead of time. Neither is necessarily right or wrong; it depends mostly on which you would prefer to do. If other family members are planning to sign up, make sure they accompany you to visit the classes. Practicing martial arts as a family is becoming more and more popular. Some schools offer family classes, where family members, regardless of age or rank, can work out together. Also, family discounts on tuition are often available.

When you discuss cost with the head instructor, make sure you know what you are getting. Can you attend unlimited classes? Some schools restrict attendance to two or three times a week. If you intend to come only two or three times a week, then this causes no problem. Ask for the instructor's policy on coming to more classes. Can you pay a little extra for the opportunity?

Be sure to ask about rank promotion tests. These are often a hidden expense. Each time you master the techniques of one belt level, and move on to the next, you generally have to take a test, either formally or informally. These tests and the new belt may (and usually do) cost money. Again, this is usual and customary, but you should be aware of the expense. Also, ask what kind of uniform and equipment are necessary. Get a general idea of the cost.

The cost for training may be anywhere from $25-70 a month. This might be slightly higher in certain areas. Testing fees can range from $25-70 for colored belts, and $100-200 for black belt testing. Only you can decide if it is worthwhile. By checking with various schools in the area, you can rule out extremely high-priced schools, but the best value isn't necessarily the cheapest school. The best school isn't necessarily the most expensive one, either.

Finally, check with the head instructor to see if you can get a free introductory lesson. Most will be happy to comply. These lessons usually last ten to fifteen minutes and introduce you to the very basic techniques that you will learn. This introductory lesson will help you understand the style and what will be expected of you.

Interviewing the head instructor

Once these steps have been accomplished, and you have narrowed your sights to one or two schools, be sure to arrange a talk with the head instructor. This does not mean arrange to pay the head instructor or sign up for classes. You are simply going to talk. A phone conversation will suffice if that is all that is possible, but meeting the head instructor before you sign up is imperative. The head instructor sets the tone for the entire school. If he or she is arrogant and impatient with you and your questions, he or she will likely still be arrogant and impatient during your training, which is not good.

When you meet with the head instructor, be certain to ask the questions you have collected on the way, questions about the size of the school or the ages of the participants. Now is the time to ask questions about the style and about the head instructor's own experience, as well as the expertise of any assistant instructors. Most instructors will talk about their own qualifications, but they may also be embarrassed to do so. They may prefer to sound humble; most martial arts instructors don't like to brag, especially to potential students. To brag sometimes means to lose face. Be specific and to the point with your questions. Ask how many years they have trained and who they have trained under. Also, ask if the school ever presents seminars or workshops on special martial arts areas or on other styles. Such learning experiences can be rewarding.

One of the most important questions to ask is about the frequency of promotion tests. Ask how long it takes to earn a black belt. For some styles, like Tae Kwon Do, one can test every two or three months. This means you can move pretty quickly through the ranks. One might expect to earn a black belt in less than three years. Karate schools usually require a little more time, closer to five years. Aikido, Judo and Jujutsu all take a little longer. The time involved doesn't matter, because your ultimate goal is health and fitness, not a black belt, but if you are told by a Judo instructor that you can earn a black belt in eighteen months, you'd better be wary. Such a belt won't mean much and the instructor's integrity is probably questionable. Such schools can't possibly be teaching the techniques correctly, and this can be dangerous, leading to injuries. Like other schools, some martial arts schools are diploma mills, and there is no benefit in that.

The best schools emphasize a combination of self-defense, fitness and mental well-being. Ask the instructor what he or she thinks is important about the martial art style being taught. If he or she says only one or two things—for instance, "you learn to fight well and win tournaments"— you might want to consider another school. If the instructor indicates that the martial arts style is well-rounded and you'll benefit in many ways, both mentally and physically, you are probably in the right place.

Following these steps can help you make one of the most important decisions to affect your personal goals. Choosing the right martial arts school can mean years of fitness and satisfaction.

Choosing the Right School
Questionnaire

The following questionnaire will help guide you through the sometimes confusing process of evaluating potential martial arts schools. Permission is given by the publisher to photocopy all or portions of the questionnaire for your personal use.

Choosing a Martial Arts Style

What kind of schools are available in your area?

What is the distance to the different schools?

Which ones are easiest and most convenient to get to?

What do you know about the different martial arts styles available in your area?

Do you have any physical limitations that might affect your ability to practice a certain martial arts style?

What amount of contact are you comfortable with?

What amount of contact does each school emphasize—no contact, light contact, medium or heavy contact? (Ask the instructors *and* students)

What is the variety of class offerings?

Will the days and times fit into your schedule?

Does the school have classes geared toward different skill levels and/or age groups? Determining Your Martial Arts Goals

How much times do you think you can or will devote to your martial arts training?

What aspects of the martial arts interest you most? The sport aspect, the culture and philosophy, self-defense, fitness and conditioning?

Are you interested in competition? Does your potential school emphasize competition?

Is getting a black belt important to you, or is staying in shape your main motivation?

Determine the Quality of Teaching

What is your impression of the head instructor?

Watch the assistant instructors as well. What is your impression of them?

Are there female instructors? Are there female black belts?

Do the instructors expect at least minimal amounts of respect and courtesy?

What are the methods of discipline used by the instructors?

Do men and women work together or are they segregated?

Do the instructors demonstrate techniques and correct incorrect techniques, or do they simply give commands?

Is an instructor always available during school hours?

Checking the Condition of the School

Is the workout area clean and well-lit?

Is there equipment and clutter in the way or is the workout area kept free of obstacles?

Is the floor suitable for working out without shoes?

Are the locker facilities kept clean and neat?

Is the equipment in good shape? (Patched equipment can be dangerous)

Are carpets or mats available for grappling or takedown techniques?

Are there adequate mirrors?

In striking schools, are there kicking targets and heavy bags?

Determining the Right Size of School

Is there enough room for everyone in the class to perform their techniques?

How many students are active in the school?

What is the average class size?

What is the instructor-per-student ratio? (In larger schools, larger classes will often have a lead instructor and several assistant instructors)

Is the head instructor a full-time martial arts teacher?

Ask the head instructor to describe the pros and cons about the size of his or her school.

Formality and Structure

How comfortable are you with formality and structure?

How comfortable are you with the level of discipline at the school?

Do children run around or are they expected to practice quietly?

Are the students courteous to each other?

Is each class taught in the same general way?

Do different instructors teach classes differently? How differently?

How important is consistency among instructors and classes to you?

How formal is the school? Will you be expected to bow to senior students and address them formally? Will you be comfortable doing this?

Checking Similarities to Other Students

Is there a wide variety of ages and physical abilities in the school?

Are any of the students your age, your condition?

Do other women attend classes? How many?

If you plan to work out with your children, is the school family-oriented?

Is the school adult-only?

Does the atmosphere seem friendly without being too casual?

Finding and Checking References

Ask other people for recommendations.

Check the Better Business Bureau and the local Chamber of Commerce.

Is the school well-established?

How long has the school been in business?

How often do injuries occur?

What is the most serious injury that has occurred?

How does the head instructor try to keep injuries under control?

Figuring Cost

How are classes paid for? By the hour, by the class, by tuition?

Can you attend unlimited classes?

Will you be expected to pay monthly or annually?

Is there a discount for paying several months or a year in advance? To compare different answers, determine how many classes you think you will attend each week, and the length of each class. Determine the approximate cost per lesson for an adequate comparison of different pricing structures. (The cost for two or three lessons a week is usually between $25 and $70 per month)

Is an introductory offer or free lesson available?

How often are rank promotions tests given?

How much do rank promotion tests cost? ($25 - $70 for colored belt test and $100 - $200 for black belt testing is average)

Instructors' Qualifications

Interview the head instructor. He or she sets the tone for the entire school. Impatient or arrogant head instructors are not the best teachers.

Ask any questions about the style that you may have.

What is the head instructor's experience?

How many years have they trained?

Who have they trained under?

Are other martial arts experts ever invited to instruct in the school (ie, seminars or workshops)?

What are the qualifications of the assistant instructors?

How long does it take to earn a black belt, with consistent effort and attendance?

What does the instructor think is most important about his/her martial arts style and school?

Index

About the Author

Jennifer Lawler is a black belt in Tae Kwon Do. She trains at New Horizons Black Belt Academy of Tae Kwon Do, in Lawrence, Kansas, under Masters Donald and Susan Booth. She also teaches Tae Kwon Do and self-defense classes. She is the author of several books, including "The Martial Arts Encyclopedia." She has published numerous articles on martial arts and women. She recently earned her Ph.D in English. She lives in Lawrence with her husband, Bret Kay, who is also a martial artist, and her daughter Jessica (plus two dogs who think they're her children).

Also Available from Turtle Press:
Teaching: The Way of the Master
Combat Strategy
The Art of Harmony
A Guide to Rape Awareness and Prevention
Total MindBody Training
1,001 Ways to Motivate Yourself and Others
Ultimate Fitness through Martial Arts
Taekwondo Kyorugi: Olympic Style Sparring
Launching a Martial Arts School
Advanced Teaching Report
Hosting a Martial Art Tournament
100 Lost Cost Marketing Ideas for the Martial Arts School
A Part of the Ribbon: A Time Travel Adventure
The Martial Arts Training Diary
The Martial Arts Training Diary for Kids
Neng Da: Super Punches
Martial Arts and the Law

For more information:
Turtle Press
PO Box 290206
Wethersfield CT 06129-206
1-800-77-TURTL
e-mail: sales@turtlepress.com

http://www.turtlepress.com